# • THE YOUNG •
# SharpMan's

## GUIDE TO

# GROOMING

A HOW–TO BOOK
FOR SHARPMEN AGES 13 & UP

THE EDITORS OF SHARPMAN.COM®

FIRST EDITION

D1366378

SHARPMAN
LOS ANGELES, CALIFORNIA

# THE YOUNG SHARPMAN'S GUIDE TO GROOMING:
## A HOW-TO BOOK FOR SHARPMEN AGES 13 & UP

by The Editors of SharpMan.com®

PUBLISHED BY:
SharpMan Press
11718 Barrington Court
No. 702
Los Angeles, CA 90049 U.S.A.
orders@sharpman.com
http://www.sharpman.com

ISBN: 0-9706600-2-2

Library of Congress Control Number: 2001096984

Printed in the United States of America

Art direction by Rowan Moore for Designland

10   9   8   7   6   5   4   3   2   1

# TABLE OF CONTENTS

**Got a grooming question?** Simply look it up in the table of contents or index of this guidebook.

**That's it.**

**No need to read the book from cover to cover.**
This guidebook is designed for use by busy guys on an as-needed basis. The answers to SharpMen's most common grooming questions are organized one after the other, as follows:

> **THE GROOMING ISSUE:**
> *The name of the grooming topic.*
>
> **THE FACTS:**
> *A brief explanation of why the grooming issue arises.*
>
> **THE GROOMING SOLUTION:**
> *Straightforward tips to meet your specific grooming need, often in a step-by-step format.*
>
> **REQUIRED GEAR:**
> *A listing of the tools required to accomplish your grooming goal.*

**And you're done.**

Looking sharp isn't about great genetics or daily workouts. The classic movie actor Humphrey Bogart probably couldn't have benched 300 and would have starved as an underwear model, but the girls loved him.

Looking sharp is about *maximizing* on *your* physical attributes. For example, your hair type and the shape of your face can help determine your best cut or facial hair option. *The Young SharpMan's Guide to Grooming* will help you capitalize on *what you've got.*

Looking sharp also means not losing on the *easy* points. Girls, school interviewers and others are turned off by mangled fingernails, overpowering cologne and poor posture. *The Young SharpMan's Guide to Grooming* will clue you in to common grooming missteps.

And don't bother reading from cover to cover. This guidebook is designed to be a handy reference for use on an as-needed basis. Simply scan the table of contents or the index to find the answer to your immediate grooming question. You'll get step-by-step tips on how to sharpen your look *fast.* We've even thrown in a list of required gear for your next trip to the store. *That's it.*

# THE GROOMING ISSUE: WASHING UP 101

## THE FACTS:

When you were a kid, avoiding the tub was like a badge of honor - he who stays dirtier longer wins. But as you moved into your teens, your mother's nagging ("Wash your face!") was joined by Mother Nature's not-so-subtle hint that you needed to wash up: acne.

*Life is cruel.* Luckily, as it turns out, keeping your skin as clear as it can be is as simple as listening to your mom.

## THE GROOMING SOLUTION:

Skin problems, types and products may vary, but the basics remain constant. The ideal skin care program includes four steps: cleansing, exfoliating, moisturizing and sun protection.

### REQUIRED GEAR

• Non-drying soap or facial cleanser.
• Light exfoliant.
• Light moisturizer.
• Sunscreen with SPF 15 or greater.

Sounds time consuming? It's not. You'll find that once you get into the habit of going through these steps, you'll easily cut your prep time to three minutes three times a day: morning, after school and before bed.

***Step One: Clean.*** Before you do anything, always ensure that your skin is clean. While most guys grab the nearest bar of soap, consider picking up a bar or cleanser that promises not to over-dry - the gentler, the better, even if you don't have "sensitive skin."

***Step Two: Scrub.*** Once your skin is clean, consider removing the patches of dead skin cells that naturally build up on the surface of your face. Doing so will help prevent blackheads and other breakouts. It is only necessary to use an exfoliant once or twice a week.

***Step Three: Lube.*** Think you don't need to moisturize? Think again. A failure to utilize this simple tool often leads SharpMen to develop itchy facial hair growth, blotchy skin and breakouts. Guys who drink a lot of caffeinated sodas, smoke cigarettes, or spend time in over-heated houses and classrooms during the winter need to lube up more than most.

Choose a moisturizer that is super light and "hypo-allergenic." Light products won't overwhelm your pores and cause breakouts. Does your skin have oily spots where you break out more often? Apply the moisturizer *around* these areas.

Moisturizing products work best when applied while your skin is still slightly damp from the shower. This helps lock in hydration.

**Step Four: Screen.** Sunscreen is your last and most important step. Yes, that means you. Even guys who only see the sun during a short morning ride to school require sun protection. A good sunscreen can make the difference between sharp-looking skin and skin that looks haggard and tired as you go from being a young SharpMan to a great-looking older SharpMan. Oh, yeah, and then there's that whole no-skin-cancer thing. A nice perk to great-looking skin. Love the way your skin looks when it's tan? See the *Safe Tanning* section of this guidebook for more information.

**Step Five: Pay attention** to changes in your skin, and adjust accordingly. If you begin to peel in the winter months, cut down on the exfoliation and up your moisturizer; if you find your skin becoming oilier in the summer months, switch to a less drying soap, exfoliate more often and go light on the moisturizer. Depending on your activities and schedule, recognize that your skin is likely to change as you get older, so stay on top of it.

**SHARPNOTE:** If you'd like to cut out a skin care step, look for a light moisturizer and sunscreen combo. Because sunscreen only lasts about an hour after application, go for the good stuff, SPF 15 or higher, to get the most for your money. Use a sunscreen-free moisturizer after your evening wash-up.

See the *Acne* section of this guidebook for more information.

# THE GROOMING ISSUE: ACNE

## THE FACTS:

Acne is a fact of life for most young SharpMen. The worst part is that it doesn't go away – despite the myth that acne ends after age 25, many SharpMen continue to break out all their lives. The good news? *You can control it.* Whether you've got a face-full or an occasional breakout, simply washing up and learning to deal with breakouts as they happen can ensure that your skin looks sharp.

### REQUIRED GEAR

- Exfoliant.
- Matches.
- Needle.
- Cotton ball.
- Alcohol.
- Tissue paper.
- Facial mud.
- Light moisturizer.

Most acne occurs in the form of whiteheads (*pustules*), blackheads, or more rarely, inflamed *papules* ("zits"). These papules are whiteheads plus bacteria.

The differences between these miseries are miniscule, but important. Normal pores produce oil, which functions as the skin's natural hydrator. When a pore becomes blocked, the oil builds up inside the pore, causing swelling and sometimes infection. Unclogging the pores is not as easy as it sounds. This is because our biggest ally – natural exfoliation – is also our biggest enemy.

*Huh?* Read on:

Your skin completely sheds itself and builds up anew every month or so. The problem is that skin sheds unevenly, leaving some new skin and other areas of dry and flaky old skin. So, while a whitehead is simply a pore blocked with your body's own hydration system, a blackhead is a whitehead that is topped off with a plug of dead skin and dirt.

These blackheads take weeks to form, so it makes sense that they don't disappear overnight. When bacteria find their way into a clogged pore, the pore becomes inflamed - red and irritated. Your body's natural defenses take over, and white blood cells flock to the area to attack the bacteria and blockage, creating a full-blown papule, or "zit."

# THE GROOMING SOLUTION:

Most acne can be reduced or eliminated by simply washing your skin in the morning, after school and before you turn in at night. See the *Washing Up 101* section of this guidebook for more information.

*Try scrubbing.* Another option for arresting the development of acne is to add a manual exfoliant to your skin care regimen. Several "scrubs" are available on the market, but beware: many of the natural scrubs contain walnut shells and other rough ingredients that can tear your pores, causing scarring and even infection. Opt for manufactured scrubs that contain smooth beads that will not damage your skin; chemical scrubs, such as those containing *alpha hydroxy acid* ("AHA") or products that utilize your own rubbing action to remove dead skin cells.

*Try washing.* If you generally break out on your forehead and around your hairline, the oil from your *hair* may be the problem. Oily hair can block pores and cause breakouts – especially when in goes unwashed for a couple of days. Make a point of washing your hair every day and washing the skin around your hairline each morning, after school and before you turn in.

*Don't touch.* In general, avoid picking at your face. Picking irritates existing acne and creates new acne by spreading bacteria. Plus, the more you pick, the more red and obvious your zits look.

*Drain properly.* If you've got a whitehead and a big week ahead of you, resist the urge to squeeze. "Popping" your blemishes causes the skin to burst unevenly, often creating bruising and an unsightly red scab.

Instead, take a quick shower to open your pores. Sterilize a small needle by holding it over a flame and *gently* puncture the top of the whitehead. Wrap a small piece of tissue paper around each of your forefingers and – *using as little force as possible* – help the puss gently ooze out of the escape valve you've created. The less you push, the less red and noticeable your former blemish will be.

Once the initial white stuff is gone, resist the urge to keep squeezing and bruise your face. Instead, clean the area with a cotton ball soaked in alcohol and apply a small dab of facial "mud," often called a facial "mask," available at most drugstores. The mud will suck out the remaining liquid and help the blemish heal overnight.

Facial mud can also help bring down blemishes that you have not drained, and is generally less drying than over-the-counter acne lotions.

The next morning, apply a small amount of light moisturizer to help the affected area heal. *Do not attempt to drain your blemishes if your skin is prone to scarring.*

**Avoid cysts.** If you develop a large, hard blemish with no whitehead, or a whitehead that fails to yield a proportionate amount of puss, *leave it alone.* You may have an acne cyst that will not respond to squeezing, but will eventually recede. Alternatively, visit a dermatologist for a faster remedy.

**Getting more help.** Of course, not all acne is the product of poor skin care; see a dermatologist if your skin does not respond to consistent cleaning.

# THE GROOMING ISSUE:
## ACNE SCARRING & PITTING

# THE FACTS:

Some teen acne leaves scarring and deep pitting long after the blemishes are gone.

# THE GROOMING SOLUTION:

If you find that your skin scars easily, refrain from picking at your blemishes to avoid further scarring.

Too late? One way to "smooth" out skin and reduce the effects of scarring is to generate new skin growth with a chemical agent that peels away the uppermost layers of the skin. As new skin develops, the appearance of top-layer scarring is reduced. Obviously, no over-the-counter product is strong enough to do this safely. If you're interested in this treatment, visit a dermatologist for a consultation on a "chemical peel" or on "laser resurfacing."

# THE GROOMING ISSUE: COLD SORES

## THE FACTS:

It's hard to feel confident with a big blister on your lip. Cold sores, often called fever blisters, are caused by a common, contagious viral infection called *herpes one*. The infection causes blisters on the lips, around the mouth and occasionally on the gums. The blisters fill with fluid, dry up and then heal over. If left untreated, a cold sore will take anywhere from four to ten days to clear up, but the virus remains in your system, often lying dormant for some time before another cold sore appears.

Stress, colds, flu, sunburn, eating certain nuts or coming in contact with someone who has an active cold sore can all cause a blister breakout. That's when your battle begins.

---

### REQUIRED GEAR

*For prevention:*
- Lip balm with SPF 15 or higher.
- Over-the-counter or prescription creams and ointments.
- Prescription oral medication.

*For treatment:*
- Over-the-counter or prescription creams, ointments and pills.

---

## THE GROOMING SOLUTION:

Your ideal solution is to arrest the breakout of a blister *before* it reaches the skin surface. Often this is possible by simply treating your lips in time.

How do you do this most effectively?

*Identify the start.* Begin by identifying the early symptoms. Most cold sore sufferers will first feel a tingling, burning or itching sensation in the area on or around their lips. While the application of an over-the-counter product may help, seeing your dermatologist for prescription medication may be more effective.

*Avoid breakouts.* Once you've been infected, as with other forms of illness, the frequency and severity of breakouts largely depend on your stress level and general health. By learning to manage your reaction to stress, you may be able to inhibit breakouts or even control the beginning of a breakout. Some physicians advise closing your eyes, breathing slowly and deeply and envisioning your blister shrinking back into your skin. At the same time, help boost your immune system by drinking fluids, eating well and getting an ample amount of sleep.

It also helps to reduce the circumstances that promote breakouts. If you feel a sore coming on, keep the affected area out of the sun by wearing a hat and a lip balm with SPF 15 or higher. Many doctors also advise patients to avoid eating nuts, a common aggravator.

**See a physician.** If your efforts to prevent a breakout prove futile, the correct treatment can speed up your healing process significantly. At the very least, you'll want to reduce the discomfort as much as possible. See a dermatologist for strong prescription medication.

**Avoid spreading.** Don't scratch or pick at your sore. Doing so may irritate the wound (prolonging the breakout) or cause the infection to spread to other areas of your lips or mouth.

If you do touch your sore, refrain from touching your eyes and face and promptly wash your hands. During and after your infection, try to change your towels, washcloths and pillowcases more frequently to avoid further spread and recurrent breakouts.

**SHARPNOTE ONE:** Can you give cold sores to someone that you kiss? Yes, but only when your cold sore is active. Kissing or sharing a soda, towel or other item with someone when you *don't* have an active sore will not infect your friends.

**SHARPNOTE TWO:** Never had a cold sore? Initial infection generally occurs when you come into contact with another infected person. For this reason, avoid kissing or otherwise coming into contact with someone who has a blister on or around their mouth. Also avoid drinking from the same glass or using the same towel as anyone with a visible sore. Note that while highly contagious, particularly at the early stage of the sore, infection is unlikely to be spread in the absence of a visible breakout.

# THE GROOMING ISSUE: COSMETIC ALTERATIONS

## THE FACTS:

While altering one's outward appearance – especially surgically – is by no means required of any SharpMan, those guys who *are* curious about doing so are no less sharp. After all, if it makes you feel better, why not?

## THE GROOMING SOLUTION:

For older SharpMen, facial surgery may be a way to look younger. For guys who are already young, surgical corrections are a way to reshape certain facial elements. For example, think your ears stick out too far? Ear pinning can tuck them in a bit closer to your hairline. Has acne left your skin looking like the surface of the moon? Laser resurfacing can smooth out the indentations of acne scarring.

The more minor facial surgery techniques are hardly "surgery" at all. Some procedures, like ear pinning, can be quickly performed after school – and have you back in class the next day. Healing time depends on you, but the localized "tender" feeling should cease within a couple of weeks.

To find out more about the variety of procedures available to young men, contact your dermatologist or physician for a referral.

**SHARPNOTE ON COSMETIC ALTERATIONS:** Deciding whether to change the way you look is a personal decision. Ultimately, the way *you* view your face, ears, nose – whatever – is far more important than the opinion of your friends or the girls you meet. After all, there are always going to be those girls who claim that they are not attracted to guys with big ears and noses. Of course, there are also many girls who claim that they are not attracted to guys who are not blonde and blue-eyed.

The point is – who cares?

It's impossible to appeal to all girls – and people – everywhere, and there *is* a lot of merit to presenting yourself as you are. If you feel comfortable with the way you look, you're bound to be much more appealing to people than if you go out and spend money on a procedure that may end up looking – well – *bad*.

In other words, *project confidence and the girls will respond.* As for those girls who can't see past what you've got – who wants them, anyway?

# THE GROOMING ISSUE: THE SHARP SHAVE

# THE FACTS:

At some point, all young SharpMen must face the razor. A few simple tips can make the difference between a great shave and a face covered with toilet tissue.

## REQUIRED GEAR

---

• Twin- or triple-blade razor.
• Shaving cream.

# THE GROOMING SOLUTION:

**Step One: *Open your pores.*** You plan to bathe, don't you? If so, you'll be taking the first step to a great shave. Go ahead and turn on the shower. A good shave requires heat to open up your pores and allow the blade's edge to do the job it was designed to do.

That's right, gentlemen, we said *blade*, so throw that electric razor in the drawer. No electric, whether black, chrome, digital or waterproof can beat a blade. Just ask your father. Chances are he never used that fancy shaving gadget you bought him last Father's Day. If he says otherwise, he's either fibbing or too old to remember the perks that come with a close shave.

**Step Two: *Prepare your tools.*** Complete your shower, allowing the steam to linger in your bathroom. Turn on the hot water – and only the hot water – in your sink and drop in your blade. Remember, *heat is your friend.* After a few minutes, add only as much cool water as you need to avoid a visit to the local burn center, and wet your face thoroughly.

**Step Three: *Apply your shaving cream.*** That's shaving *cream.* Not foam. Not gel. If the contents are under pressure, for a few dollars more, you can do better. But whatever product you choose, be careful to apply it to only those areas that you intend to shave. The outline you create will be your guide, and when all is gone, you'll know you're done.

**Step Four: *Pick up your blade*** and start with the side opposite to your dominant hand. In other words, if you are right-handed, start with the left side of your face. This is the easiest part of your shave and, given the fact that your eyes are generally half-glued shut in the morning, you'll be less likely to scar yourself. Most young SharpMen fear blades because few enjoy seeing their own blood in the morning. To avoid this, use long, smooth, consistent strokes over your face, with just enough pressure to prevent the blade from snagging, but not so much that you gouge your skin.

Your strokes should run the blade down your cheek. That's *down*, not up, and not sideways. It's remarkable how many men still believe that a close shave requires going "against the grain." Shaving is like painting a wood fence: go with the grain, always. Any other way, and you run the risk of irritating your skin.

If you aren't satisfied with the closeness of your shave, simply change blades. Most twin- or triple-blade razors will do the job for five to ten days, depending on the strength of your growth. If your shave is not as close as you would like, or your current blade begins to feel rough against your skin, then it's time to discard the blade and pick up a new one.

**Step Five: Rinse.** Place your blade back under the warm water after every three strokes, and, when finished, rinse your face thoroughly. This last step is important, not only for the obvious goal of removing lingering cream, but because it's a fast way to check your work. If you feel any missed stubble as you rinse, just pick up your blade and touch up.

**Step Six: Gently pat your face dry.** Don't rub. If you use cologne or aftershave, apply it first to your body; whatever is still left on your hands is more than enough for your freshly shaven skin.

**SHARPNOTE ON SHAVING CUTS:** Available for a couple of dollars at your local drugstore, styptic sticks or "pencils" quickly stop the bleeding associated with shaving cuts and nicks.

To use a styptic stick, first blot away any excess blood with a tissue. Wet the tip of the stick and apply the wet edge to your cut by dabbing the area gently. As the watered-down material dries on your skin, a white chalky outline will appear. When this matted powder has dried completely, simply wipe away the obvious white stuff around your cut or nick with a damp tissue. For minor cuts, only one application is required. For bigger blunders, a couple of swipes may be required before you can safely exit the bathroom.

# THE GROOMING ISSUE: AVOIDING RAZOR BURN

## THE FACTS:

For some, shaving is like going into battle – a battle against "razor burn," an irritation that develops when sensitive skin becomes irritated by shaving. By simply doing a bit of prep-work before your shave, your chances of coming out without a burn are greatly enhanced. On the other hand, if you jump into battle with no protection, your skin will suffer the fiery consequences.

### REQUIRED GEAR

• Shaving cream.
• Twin- or triple-blade razor.
• Moisturizing aftershave.
• Tweezers.
• Rubbing alcohol.

## THE GROOMING SOLUTION:

Although it sounds tedious, protecting your skin from the shaving battle-ground is easier than you think. Dermatologists recommend a simple regimen of preparing the skin, choosing super-sensitive tools, and following up with a moisturizing aftershave. Even in extreme cases, simple over-the-counter products can help heal the most severe razor burn.

*Step One: Prepare for the fight.* Most young SharpMen assume that avoiding razor burn requires the exclusive use of an electric razor – and the chance of missing out on a close shave. Not so. Simply showering before you shave will properly prepare your hair follicles and pores for a razor-burn-free shave and minimize existing irritation. For more information, see *The Sharp Shave* section of this guidebook.

*Step Two: Choose a moisturizing shaving cream* for your morning ritual. The more creamy your shaving product, the less likely you will be to develop dry-skin related irritation. As you shave, don't skimp on the shaving cream; to avoid razor burn, make sure your entire shaving area is lathered. Then, when shaving, angle your razor *with* the grain, pointed down, to prevent causing further irritation or ingrown hairs.

Don't press the razor too firmly on your skin. Gentle pressure is enough. Take your time and pay attention to the task at hand.

**Step Three: Soothe your skin.** After you've finished shaving, take a moment to be good to it. Splashing warm water on freshly shaven skin will close your pores and help prevent irritation. Following up with a moisturizing aftershave balm will do much more. Moisturizing aftershaves disinfect and add a bit more moisture to protect sensitive skin — particularly in those dry winter months when skin becomes more sensitive to shaving.

**Step Four: Treat the wounds.** If all the prep work in the world won't protect your skin from razor burn, moisturizing aftershave treatments containing *tea tree extract*, a natural ingredient that calms burns and prevents the build-up of irritating dead skin cells and ingrown hairs, are your best defense. Simply apply a small amount after you rinse off your shaving cream.

Do your facial hairs grow back into your skin — causing a red, raised spot that looks like a zit from far away? These are called *ingrown hairs*, and they can be avoided. Before using any aftershave product, gently press on the raised area. This will cause shallow ingrown hairs to pop out. Remove more deeply embedded hairs with a pair of *clean* tweezers. Before using tweezers, always clean the tip with rubbing alcohol to sanitize and prevent unattractive infections on your face. To prevent tweezer pain, numb the area with an ice cube or over-the-counter numbing agent before hair removal.

**SHARPNOTE:** When buying a shaving aid, be sure to grab a *cream*, not a gel. Creams provide more moisture and offer better protection against razor burn.

# THE GROOMING ISSUE: FACIAL HAIR OPTIONS

# THE FACTS:

If you have enough growth, facial hair can make a strong statement, in addition to making you look older. Better still, experimenting with facial hair can give you and your skin a break from the daily shave routine – a plus for young SharpMen with sensitive skin.

# THE GROOMING SOLUTION:

Before you make the move to the hairy side, consider your various facial hair options:

*Sideburns.* Sideburns are easy to grow and maintain. But realize: despite the recent upsurge in popularity for long, thick sideburns, your ideal length and width depends largely on the shape of *your* face and what looks best on you.

*Goatee.* The various goatee styles are all kid-brother versions of the full beard. They cover the chin area, but do not extend down beyond the jaw line. Because less facial hair area is required, goatees are relatively easy to grow and are ideal for young SharpMen with patchy growth. Of course, all this comes at a price; consistent shaving and trimming are required to maintain that distinctive look. Goatees can be worn with or without a matching mustache. Mini-goatees, also known as "jazz dots," are also popular.

*Mustache.* That tuft of hair above the upper lip has many variations, is relatively easy to grow and requires very little maintenance. Most young SharpMen may find that a neat, short mustache is their best bet.

*Full beard.* The full beard covers the chin, jaw line and upper lip. While less common for young SharpMen, beards are easy to grow and ideal for masking scars and other skin or structural imperfections. Beards generally require a strong, full growth, but longer beard styles can cover patchy or uneven growth. Of course, having half of your face covered in hair is a pretty strong statement. Experimenting with this style will let you know if you can carry it off.

*Combo styles.* The combinations of mustaches, goatees and side-burns are unlimited and can be flattering. Of course, the more complicated your chosen design, the more shaving and trimming maintenance work it will require.

**SHARPNOTE:** Recognize that — however small — all facial hair styles make a statement. Despite your personality, growing some styles of facial hair will make people see you differently. Sometimes in a good way — and sometimes in a bad way. All men are judged by the image they project — whether "clean cut" (even if they are not) or "bad" (even if they never have been). So choose the look you cultivate carefully — as you will be judged and treated different-ly based on it.

See the *Choosing Facial Hair to Flatter the Shape of Your Face* section of this guidebook for more information.

# THE GROOMING ISSUE: Choosing Facial Hair to Flatter the Shape of Your Face

# THE FACTS:

Looking sharp is all about maximizing on what you *have*. If you are interested in experimenting with facial hair, simply taking the shape of your face and other features into consideration before choosing a style can cut out a lot of your guess work and yield great results.

# THE GROOMING SOLUTION:

Match the general shape of your face and facial features to one of the following:

*Long, thin face.* Young SharpMen with long, thin faces look great when they fill out the look of their faces. If you're one of those, avoid longer goatees, as they will add to the length to your chin. Instead, try a short pair of sideburns to round out your jaw line. This style will draw attention away from the lower half of your face. For those who choose to and can grow beards, keep them trimmed very tightly around the chin and leave the sides fuller.

*Round, full face.* Guys with round faces can look "pudgy," even if their bodies are not. Often lengthening the look of your face can help. Try a goatee – goatees draw the eye to a point at the chin and make jaws look less full. Avoid narrow mustaches and any hair on the jaw line – these styles only add to the roundness of your face.

*Small chin.* Young SharpMen with small chins – also called "weak chins" – look great when they beef up this area of the face. A fuller goatee can do wonders for drawing out your chin. Avoid mustaches without beards, as they will tend to overshadow your chin and bring you back to square one.

*Covering scarring.* Facial hair is an excellent way to cover scars, but keep in mind that your hair cover should nonetheless suit the shape of your face. Even for guys with substantial acne scarring, a tightly trimmed beard or goatee can work just as well as the full job. For best results, grow the full beard first, mark the area you'd like to mask and style accordingly.

**SHARPNOTE:** If you are prone to acne breakouts due to oily skin, realize that while facial hair may cover your breakouts, it may also make them worse. The added oils around facial hair may further block pores, causing more common and lengthier breakouts. Before covering acne with facial hair, consider treating the source. See the *Washing Up 101* and *Acne* sections of this guidebook for more information.

# THE GROOMING ISSUE:
## GROWING FACIAL HAIR 101

# THE FACTS:

Once you've decided to grow facial hair, simply following a few easy steps will ensure that you are able quickly determine which look is most flattering to you, with minimal re-growth time.

# THE GROOMING SOLUTION:

**Step One: Timing is everything.**
If possible, begin your experiment while on vacation or during a school break. This way, if you feel self-conscious or would like to alter your new look, you can choose to be out-of-sight during the transition. Another good reason to grow facial hair while out of school? Those first few weeks can look pretty unkempt - much more suited to time at the beach or lake than a day in class.

## REQUIRED GEAR

• Twin- or triple-blade razor.
• Electric beard trimmer.
• Beard trimming scissors and comb.
• Moisturizing aftershave with tea tree extract.

**Step Two: Do nothing.** Stop shaving and leave your face alone for about three weeks. Sounds simple, doesn't it? It's not. There's always a temptation to start trimming and shaping as soon as your hair gets past the stubble stage. Fight the urge. Trimming and shaping too early can result in removing too much hair in some places. The result? A longer wait, a style unsuited to your face, or frustration resulting in an early end to the experiment.

**Step Three: Choose a shape.** Once you have enough hair to work with, you can begin shaping your facial hair. If you are uncertain about what you want, make a list of all of the styles you like, beginning with the styles that require the most amount of hair (i.e., a full beard) and ending with those that require the least (i.e., a "jazz dot"). Tailor your list to the amount of facial hair you are able to grow. Then begin experimenting with the styles at the beginning of your list. Give yourself a few days to test out each look before moving on to the next one. This way you'll have the opportunity to try out several different styles with a minimum of re-growth time in between. After all, it is easier to shave off hair than to grow back a gap you don't want.

**Step Four: Get professional help.**  Once you've chosen your basic style, visiting an old-fashioned men's barber shop may help you refine the look. That's right; skip the trendy hair salon and head for that hole-in-the-wall where your mom used to take you for haircuts. Those old guys *really* know facial hair. Ask your new barber to set the "lines" of your new look – after that, maintenance will be as easy as following his outline.

Otherwise, get yourself a good pair of beard-trimming scissors and a comb. Use a twin- or triple-blade razor to define your look and use the comb and scissors to trim your hair to the desired length. Take your time and trim gradually until you hit upon the style you want. Alternatively, save time by investing in an inexpensive electric beard trimmer with various length settings. Electric beard trimmers are available at most drugstores.

**SHARPNOTE:** Itching is a common problem in the first few weeks of facial hair growth. To minimize itching, wash your face thoroughly and use a light moisturizer. Moisturizing aftershaves containing a natural ingredient called *tea tree extract* do double-duty: they moisturize *and* prevent the development of ingrown hairs.

See the *Facial Hair Maintenance* section of this guidebook for specific information on trimming and shaping.

# THE GROOMING ISSUE: FACIAL HAIR MAINTENANCE

## THE FACTS:

If you've gone to the trouble of growing out your facial hair, picking up a couple of trimming and maintenance tricks can go a long way towards ensuring your facial hair always looks sharp.

## THE GROOMING SOLUTION:

*Ideal maintenance.* Once you've chosen your facial hair style and established the basic maintenance "lines," always trim and groom *outside* of those lines.

*Keeping clean.* To keep facial hair clean, use the same shampoo you use for the hair on your head and rinse thoroughly. For young SharpMen with dry skin or course facial hair, using a small amount of hair conditioner will keep skin from flaking and tough facial hair from scarring the girls.

### REQUIRED GEAR

- Electric beard trimmer.
- A wide-toothed (beards) or narrow-toothed (all other styles) comb.
- A small pair of sharp scissors.

*Using a beard trimmer.* While it is possible to use scissors and a comb, an inexpensive electric beard trimmer will prove to be your best facial hair maintenance equipment. The various trimmer settings will help you quickly maintain and even out facial hair length (read: no bald spots), in addition to helping you define and maintain a clean neckline. Electric beard trimmers are available at most drugstores.

*Combing out.* Once you've cleaned and trimmed your facial hair, take a moment to quickly comb it into place. A narrow-toothed comb is ideal for mustaches, goatees and sideburns. Why not use your hairbrush? A comb has the added advantage of allowing you to easily isolate and trim unwanted hair as you go.

*Trimming tips for goatees.* Goatee styles come and go. Fad is less important than finding a style that suits the shape of your face and maintaining it properly. In most cases, simply keeping your goatee short, clean and neat goes a long way. Shave around the ideal shape of the goatee, always on the *outside* of the line, and follow up with a quick scissor trim or an electric beard trimmer to maintain the length.

**Trimming tips for mustaches.** Keep your mustache trimmed above your upper lip to avoid being one of those guys who constantly has food caught in his facial hair. When trimming your mustache, begin by trimming from the middle and work your way out to each side.

**Trimming tips for beards.** Beards look best when kept tight and well trimmed. To avoid a sloppy look, shave any hair below your jaw line every three or four days, depending on how aggressive your growth is. You can make this job easier by using an electric beard trimmer. The upper line of a beard is generally not shaved, unless you feel that the natural line of your beard is too high.

**Trimming tips for other styles.** Nearly all facial hair styles require you to shave and trim to avoid looking sloppy. Depending on your chosen style, you may prefer to use a beard trimmer to maintain the length of the hair and a razor for areas that require a clean shave.

For information on trimming your sideburns, see the *Making Your Haircut Last* section of this guidebook.

# THE GROOMING ISSUE: TRAINING FACIAL HAIR

# THE FACTS:

For years SharpMen have "trained" their facial hair into totally unnatural – but then-fashionable – growth patterns. Think of the handlebar mustache or other gravity-defying facial hair styles. You think those hairs weren't coaxed?

Historically men have used mustache wax or paste, a small mustache comb and their fingers to coax facial hair into the desired style. Today's young SharpMen can apply this technique to facial hair that grows at odd angles.

# THE GROOMING SOLUTION:

*Training products.* To train your facial hair, choose a can of mustache wax or one of the many pomades, waxes and gels currently available on the market for head hair. The key is to find a product strong enough to hold your hair, but one that does not irritate your skin. Young SharpMen with oily skin may prefer a super-hold gel to avoid breakouts, while dry-haired SharpMen may wish to use a pomade to prevent flaking. When in doubt, ask your barber or hairstylist for a recommendation.

### REQUIRED GEAR

• Pomade, gel or wax.
• Narrow-toothed mustache comb.

*Training techniques.* Once you've chosen your product, simply apply a small amount to your palm and then a smaller amount to your facial hair. *Use less than you think you need* – adding is a lot easier than washing out and starting over. Once you've applied your gel, pomade or wax, use a narrow-toothed comb to shape your hair, using the hair product as the "adhesive." Keep this up and your hair should eventually give in.

# THE GROOMING ISSUE:
## DEALING WITH EAR & NOSE HAIR

## THE FACTS:

Ever wake up one morning and discover a stray hair making its way out of your ear or nostril? Beware the tentacles of terror – they look gross.

Young SharpMen don't just *suddenly* sprout nose hair – it's always been there. Tiny ear and nose hairs act as barriers that protect the body from airborne dirt and pollen, the same way lashes protect the eye. As SharpMen get older, changing hormonal levels affect hair growth. The male hormone *dihydrotestosterone* (DHT), the culprit behind male pattern baldness, may also be linked to nasal and ear hair growth. This explains why women don't commonly experience similar problems. Although researchers have established that increased levels of DHT are responsible for scalp hair loss, the exact relationship of DHT to nasal and ear hair is unclear.

> ## REQUIRED GEAR
>
> ————
>
> • Small blunt-nosed scissors, *or*
> • Electric ear and nose hair trimmer.

## THE GROOMING SOLUTION:

Ever heard that trimming ear or nose hair causes it to grow back thicker? It's not true. Trimming unwanted hair does not cause more hair to grow. So feel free to trim any hair that doesn't suit your sense of style. But when we say trim, we mean *trim*. *Do not pluck*. Not only does plucking hurt, it may cause a tearing of the skin on the inside your nose, which can lead to redness, swelling and infection.

To trim nose and ear hair, use a small pair of blunt-nosed scissors to carefully shorten your hairs. It is not necessary to trim too closely. Simply cut down those hairs that protrude from your nose and ears.

Alternatively, use an ear and nose hair trimmer, a small electric or battery-operated device that uses a rotating or oscillating blade to quickly and safely trim hair. Both mechanisms work well, although the oscillating blade is often considered less painful.

**SHARPNOTE:** Trimmers are safe to use, so long as you refrain from forcing them too far into your nasal cavity or ear canal. Always review the instructions before going where no man has gone before.

# THE GROOMING ISSUE: TAMING THE "UNIBROW"

## THE FACTS:

Having one long eyebrow span the area over both eyes makes some young SharpMen uncomfortable. Why? In general, contemporary men's grooming ideals dictate that eyebrows connected by a patch of hair look less polished than two distinct eyebrow lines.

## THE GROOMING SOLUTION:

Young SharpMen have several options for removing the unwanted hair in between their eyebrows. The method you choose will largely depend on the strength of your eyebrow hair, your budget and your willingness to maintain your eyebrows on a regular basis.

### REQUIRED GEAR

- Slant-nosed metal tweezers.
- Pencil or straight edge.
- Alcohol or other antiseptic.
- Cotton balls.

*Tweezing.* While hardly pleasurable, using a pair of slant-nosed metal tweezers to pluck the hair in between your eyebrows is often your easiest and least expensive option. You can tweeze in the privacy of your own bathroom and remove stray hairs as they reappear. See below for step-by-step tips on safely plucking your unibrow.

Alternatively, consider visiting a professional for the initial grunt work. He or she will shape your brows and instruct you on maintaining your new look. Most aestheticians (professionals once known as "beauticians") who service women also accept male clients. Ask your barber or hairstylist for a referral.

*Waxing.* Wax treatments involve spreading hot or cold wax over the area targeted for hair removal, placing a strip of cloth over the wax, rubbing vigorously and then ripping the cloth – along with the wax and the hair – in one smooth stroke. Waxing removes the hair and hair root, and is generally considered to be longer-lasting than plucking, because your roots take several weeks to reestablish themselves. While more painful than plucking, waxing takes only seconds and the sting disappears quickly.

Although there are many home waxing kits that allow SharpMen to wax their own unibrows, consider going to a professional salon for this treatment. First-time home waxers have been known to injure themselves or wax off more hair than intended. *Oops.*

As with plucking, most aestheticians who service women also accept male clients. Ask your barber or hairstylist for a referral.

*Electrolysis & Laser.* While less common among young SharpMen, electrolysis and laser hair removal treatments are two additional – and substantially more expensive – options for removing hair between your eyebrows. For more information on these techniques, see the *Removing Back Hair* section of this guidebook.

*Maintenance.* Even if you regularly visit a professional salon to have your unibrow cured, you will always need to do some home maintenance for stray hairs. Similarly, if your unibrow is not full enough to require a trip to the salon, consider the following tips for grooming and shaping your eyebrows:

*Pluck just out of the shower.* It is easier and less painful to tweeze hairs when you first get out of the shower, as the heat and steam will have opened your pores and loosened their grip on the hairs.

*Map out your route.* Where should each eyebrow begin and end? Hold a pencil or other straight edge against the end of your nose, straight up to your eyebrow. Your inner brow should begin where the pencil meets your brow and end about a quarter of an inch past the outer corner of your eye.

*Removing hair.* Grasping the tweezers with your thumb and forefinger, firmly grab and pluck away from your face using a single forceful movement. Only attempt to pluck one hair at a time to minimize pain. Refrain from picking at hairs too short for easy plucking to avoid breaking the skin.

*Stop to assess.* As you pluck, try to keep your work balanced. The last thing you want is for one eyebrow to be thinner or shorter than the other. For this reason, alternate plucking each brow every few hairs and watch the balance between the two.

*Don't over-pluck.* Pluck slowly and take away only those stray hairs that are particularly obvious. When in doubt, stop plucking. No SharpMan wants to be the guy with eyebrows that are too "done."

*Clean up.* When you've finished tweezing, wipe the area with an alcohol-soaked cotton ball to clean and close your pores.

**SHARPNOTE:** If you've spent money on a professional, let him or her determine the "line" of your eyebrows, and then only pluck *outside* of this line.

# THE GROOMING ISSUE: EAR CARE 101

# THE FACTS:

Most SharpMen don't think about ear maintenance until they hear complaints from their T.V.-watching buddies: "Turn that down; are you deaf or something?" This exchange is usually followed by a brief – but fleeting – thought about ear cleaning. In reality, most guys refrain from cleaning their ears because they (a) don't know how, and (b) may have heard that cleaning ears improperly could lead to hearing damage.

## REQUIRED GEAR

- Soap.
- Washcloth.
- Cotton swabs.

# THE GROOMING SOLUTION:

Think it's time to clean your ears? If so, recognize that not all ear wax should be removed.

Ear wax is important: it serves as the cleaning mechanism of the ear canal. It traps dust in the inner canal and then removes the dust (along with itself) to the outer ear – the part you can reach into with your finger.

For this reason, there's no point in reaching in and digging out the build-up in your inner ear. In most cases, this mass of wax will make its own way out. It is a good idea to clean out the opening of the ear (the part that protrudes from your head), *but stop there*. Just use a wash-cloth and mild soap to clean the outer ear while you shower. This is the *only* part of your ear you should ever touch with a cotton swab.

As for using cotton swabs, avoid sticking them into your ear canal far as they'll reach. This pushes more wax into the ear than it removes. You also run the risk of scratching the ear canal or even damaging your ear drum. Use a fresh side of the cotton swab for each of your ears.

Sometimes excess wax does accumulate in your ear. Often, this occurs because you've been too zealous with your cotton swab and crammed the wax back into your ear canal. This build-up is most safely removed by an ear nose and throat ("ENT") physician. Home kits are also available for occasional use, but should never be used before having your ears examined by a physician.

# THE GROOMING ISSUE:
## COMBATING BAD BREATH

# THE FACTS:

Most young SharpMen may not realize the strong connection between failing to floss and stinky breath. Anytime you eat or drink, small particles of food lodge themselves between your teeth. What's that? You say that you *always* brush? Brushing removes only those particles of food that lie on the *surface* of your teeth, whereas food and other smelly substances trapped between the teeth just sit there – rotting – *almost as if you had never bothered to brush at all.* The result is some seriously stinky breath.

## REQUIRED GEAR

- Waxed floss "string" for teeth spaced close together.
- Waxed floss "tape," also known as "dental tape" for teeth with gaps between them.
- Mouthwash or breath mints.
- Parsley or oral products containing parsley.

# THE GROOMING SOLUTION:

If you believe your mouth is a party to this level of stink, then flossing is for you. The following quick flossing tips will help you do the job without damaging your gums:

**Step One: Floss before you brush.** This way you ensure that the particles you removed from in between your teeth are brushed and rinsed away.

**Step Two: Use enough floss.** Use approximately 12 to 18 inches of floss and wind an end of the floss around the middle finger of each hand, leaving roughly one inch of floss between the fingertips.

**Step Three: Saw gently.** Use a gentle sawing motion to insert floss just in between your teeth-but be careful not to jerk the floss "knife" into your gums.

*Step Four: Bend as you saw.* Slowly bring the floss towards the gum line, then bend the floss on both sides, so that it curves into a "c" shape against the sides of your tooth. Use an up-and-down scraping motion to remove plaque just beneath the gum line and in between teeth.

*Step Five: Repeat.* Repeat step four on the next tooth, between all of your teeth and behind your molars, as well. Use a different one-inch portion of the floss each time you floss.

**SHARPNOTE:** Ever come in contact with a coffee-drinker or garlic-eater who doesn't realize he's wilting the greenery around him? Because it's not always possible to brush and floss after you eat and drink, arming your pocket or locker with a few tricks of the good-breath trade can be helpful when you're away from home:

*Coffee stink.* "Shallow" bad breath, such as coffee stink, only affects your tongue and mouth. These superficial bad breath brands can be easily combated with mints or mouthwash.

*Food stink.* And if you had garlic or onions for lunch or dinner? Garlic and other food smells emanate from your *digestive system*, not your mouth, so no number of mints will be enough to mask the odor for longer than the mint is in your mouth. The age-old remedy for neutralizing digestive odors is *parsley*. Ever wonder why it's always on the edge of your plate? It isn't just for garnish. So go ahead and munch on the green stuff at the end of your meal. Alternatively, most drugstores stock parsley pills for easy locker or pocket access after meals.

# THE GROOMING ISSUE: TEETH WHITENING

# THE FACTS:

Teeth can become stained for a number of reasons, the most common being consumption of sodas, coffee, tea, berries, fruit juices, smoking, certain antibiotics used to combat acne and just plain-old *life*. In other words, simply being a normal human being can cause your teeth to yellow.

The good news is that stained teeth can be safely whitened or bleached.

# THE GROOMING SOLUTION:

When considering whether to whiten your teeth, skip the infomercials and visit your dentist. He or she will check out your mouth to ensure that it's healthy enough to bleach safely and to determine whether cosmetic whitening is appropriate for you.

**Who can bleach?** Some teeth bleach better than others. Yellow teeth generally respond to treatment, while brownish or grayish teeth (caused by the use of the antibiotic *tetracycline*) are unlikely to bleach well. In some cases porcelain veneers or dental bonding may be more suitable. A dental consultation is particularly important for young SharpMen with fillings or crowns.

**Safety first.** Is bleaching gel safe? The most common active ingredient in bleaching gel is ten percent *carbamide peroxide*, which breaks down into three percent *hydrogen peroxide* when dispensed. It's been used for years and is considered safe, *especially under a dentist's supervision.*

**It's a go.** If your dentist determines that cosmetic bleaching is for you, he or she will make impressions of your teeth and create custom mouth guard trays for you. To protect your sensitive gum tissue, he or she will leave a slight space between the tray and your gums when forming the tray.

*The how-tos.* Depending on your particular discoloration and gum sensitivity, your dentist will instruct you on the proper use of your mouth guards and bleaching gel. Treatments generally last between one week to one month. Your dentist will also likely ask you to come in for a reevaluation during your treatment to ensure that your bleaching is progressing safely.

*Use in moderation.* Avoid using more gel or wearing your mouth guards longer than your dentist recommends. If you experience any pain in your teeth or gums, contact your dentist immediately.

*Side effects.* The most common side effect associated with bleaching is tooth sensitivity. Generally, this side effect is mild and temporary, lasting only as long as your bleaching treatment. Gum irritation is uncommon and generally associated with improper use of the guard trays.

*Repeat customers.* The effects of cosmetic bleaching should last indefinitely, that is, so long as you avoid staining foods and beverages and maintain good oral health. That means brushing at least twice a day, flossing, and visiting your dentist every six months for a thorough cleaning and check-up.

On the other hand, if you continue to ingest those items that stained your teeth in the first place, your teeth *will* gradually yellow again. Luckily, it's safe to repeat bleaching under a dentist's supervision.

**SHARPNOTE:** Many over-the-counter whitening toothpastes can *slowly* help remove surface stains and keep yellowing from returning once you've had it bleached away. Unfortunately, on their own, whitening toothpastes will not yield the quick, dramatic changes found with bleaching.

## SHAMPOOING 101

### SHARPCUTS
Better Cuts for Your Hair Type
Better Cuts for Your Face Type

### SHARPHAIR MAINTENANCE
Making Your Cut Last
Hair Junk
Combating Frizz
Straightening Curly Hair
Long Hair Care
Dealing with Dandruff
Date & Interview Hair

# THE GROOMING ISSUE: Shampooing 101

## THE FACTS:

In general, hair comes in three types: oily, dry or damaged. Each of these require young SharpMen to wash and condition their hair differently in order to achieve the best results.

## THE GROOMING SOLUTION:

*Oily hair.* If you find your hair to be generally oily or greasy, avoid running your hands through your hair. Despite how suave the gesture, simply putting your hands in contact with your hair transfers oil from your skin, adding oil to an already slick surface.

When it comes to washing oily hair, the drill is simple: read the front of your shampoo bottle. Choose shampoos designed specifically for oily – or "smooth" – hair. On the other hand, despite the "rinse and repeat" instruction on the back, only shampoo your hair once and skip the conditioner. If you find that your hair requires a bit of moisture in the winter months, limit conditioning to a once-a-week treatment.

> ### REQUIRED GEAR
>
> - Shampoo for your hair type.
> - Conditioner for your hair type.

*Dry hair.* If your hair doesn't feel oily in between washes and tends to look frazzled at the ends, it may require a bit of moisture. This is especially true for guys who spend a lot of time in the water or in the sun. Sure, it may look ratty to you, but dry and brittle hair is easy to manage.

To care for dry, coarse hair, find a shampoo specifically designed for this hair type. Because dry hair requires a natural build-up of scalp oil to keep it looking good, only use your dry hair shampoo every *couple* of days. Go ahead and shower daily, but skip the hair wash. On the other hand, use a good conditioner *every time* you shower – whether you shampoo or not. It may sound strange, but simply letting conditioner sit on wet, unwashed hair for a few minutes will make styling your locks that much easier.

*Damaged hair.* Young SharpMen who try to torque up their looks with bleaching or color treatments can inadvertently damage their hair. Color, bleach and similar products are pretty harsh. Drugstore home treatments are even worse. For this reason, consider splurging on a professional color or bleaching treatment. Products used by the pros are easier on hair, and professional stylists are less likely to damage your hair by keeping the product on too long.

For washing at home, ask your hairstylist to recommend a shampoo specially designed for color- or bleach-treated hair. You'll find that these products make your hair look shinier, assist in styling and maintain the color much longer than other shampoos. Of course, better-lasting color means you thrash your hair less often and save money on fewer repeat treatments.

Another way to lengthen the time between treatments is to find a "color enhancing" shampoo. These shampoos actually add your preferred color as you use them.

Because color is so tough on hair, follow your shampoo with a conditioning treatment designed for color-treated or damaged hair.

**SHARPNOTE:** Is it necessary to spring for expensive salon shampoos and conditioners for hair that is not color-treated or bleached? Not really. Often you'll find that your hair responds just as well to drugstore brands.

# THE GROOMING ISSUE:
## MATCHING YOUR CUT TO YOUR HAIR TYPE

# THE FACTS:

We've all had them: the bad haircut and the ensuing bad hair day (or *month*). Consider the connection between the two and avoid both by picking a style that suits your type of hair. That's right; long before you step up to the barber's chair, you can determine what haircuts will best flatter your type of hair.

# THE GROOMING SOLUTION:

*Straight hair.* Straight hair often lacks the volume to support high altitude hairstyles. For this reason, a simple cut is your best bet. Try a 1940s style with hair cropped short on the sides and back, front parted to the side. Avoid "cookie-cutter" haircuts, where the hair on the back and sides of your head is cut above the hairline. Helpful styling products for straight hair? Try a "volumizing" mousse or gel designed to give more bang to your straight hair buck.

*Light to medium curly hair.* While less problematic than super-curls, light to medium curls require special attention. The sides and back should be short and tight, with the hair cut above the ears. The less curl in your hair, the longer you can go with your cut on top. But avoid letting all that length go to your head. Growing your hair too long on the top and sides can leave you looking like a poodle. Too long in the back and you'll be back in the early 1980s – but not in a good way.

## REQUIRED GEAR

- *Straight hair:* volumizing mousse or gel.
- *Light to medium curly hair:* pomade, soft setting or strong hold gel.
- *Super curly hair:* setting gel.
- *Fine or thinning hair:* volumizing mousse or gel.
- Blow-dryer.

To define your curls and avoid frizz, try a soft setting gel. To control and style without curl definition, use a strong gel or pomade. With a quarter-sized amount of either product in your palm, rub hands together and apply, working into the hair with your fingertips.

*Super curly hair.* There are many casual ways to wear super-curly hair, such as the "afro," long tresses on all or two sides, or dread-locks. For a cut that won't scare the ladies, one strong style stands out for turbo-curly hair: cut hair one-fourth of an inch short all over, so that your entire head of hair is one length. Never comb out longer curly hair to avoid frizz.

To reproduce this look at home, ask your hairstylist to recommend a setting gel. With a quarter-sized amount of the product in your palm, rub hands together and apply, working into hair with your fingertips.

*Fine hair.* Fine hair can appear fuller if styled correctly. Request a short cut that pushes your hair forward. This allows each hair to cover more of your scalp, thereby making your hair look thicker than it is. Avoid cuts that call for you to comb hair sideways or back, as they highlight the fact that your hair is fine.

When styling, thicken hair by applying a half-dollar sized amount of volumizing mousse or gel to your entire head of hair. Work the product through your hair with your hands. Using a medium-heat blow-dryer, blow hair in all directions until dry, thereby giving the appearance of fuller, thicker hair.

For more information on using styling products, see the *Using Hair Junk* section of this guidebook.

**SHARPNOTE ONE:** Great hair days begin with great haircuts and practice. Take time to get to know your hair and what it can and can't do. Don't fight Mother Nature – go with what you have naturally so that your style won't look "strained." Remember that men have no mandate to change hairstyles with the seasons. Find and stick to what works for you.

**SHARPNOTE TWO:** A common misconception dictates that blow-drying is required for a great hair day. Blow-dryers are not always necessary. For shorter hairstyles, towel dry first, then apply your hair product and allow the hair to dry naturally. Don't plug in unless the product instructions call for it.

# THE GROOMING ISSUE:
## MATCHING YOUR CUT TO YOUR FACE

# THE FACTS:

In addition to matching your haircut to your hair type (see the *Matching Your Cut to Your Hair Type* section of this guidebook for more information), matching your cut to the shape of your face or those facial features you'd like to downplay is another way to get more bang for your hairstyle buck.

# THE GROOMING SOLUTION:

*Round faces.* To de-emphasize your round baby face, consider a style that moves hair away from your mug. Avoid cuts that require full hair on the sides. To add length and height to your face, choose a style with longer hair on top.

*Thin faces.* To make your face look fuller and avoid a long, thin look, skip the hairstyles with "height." Instead, speak to your hairstylist about a cut that is fuller on the sides.

*Protruding ears.* To take attention away from large or protruding ears, speak to your hairstylist about a cut that is longer on the sides. Fuller styles that creep up over the ears look best, if the shape of your face allows.

*Substantial noses.* If you feel self-conscious about your nose, avoid super-short cuts, as these tend to draw attention to all strong features.

*Facial scars.* If you'd like to mask scarring at the top or sides of your face, your hairstylist may be able to recommend a cut and style to obscure this feature. For centrally located scarring, consider one of several facial hair styles. See the *Choosing Facial Hair to Flatter the Shape of Your Face* section of this guidebook for more information. Neither option suits your style? Just ignore your scarring and you'll find that most everyone else will eventually do the same.

**SHARPNOTE:** Ready for a big change? Going from long to short hair can be a bit drastic. By the same token, gradually going from short to sloppy to long can be excruciatingly slow. How can you ease these transitions?

*Short to long.* To avoid looking sloppy during your short-to-long transition, consider growing the top part of your hair before growing out the sides.

*Long to short.* If you'd like to shorten your hair but aren't sure what length or look you'll ultimately settle on, try cutting in stages.

# THE GROOMING ISSUE:
## MAKING YOUR HAIRCUT LAST

# THE FACTS:

Man, is it time for another haircut already? It seems like just the other week you were taking time out of your schedule to get a trim and fork out the cash. Take heart. With a few SharpMan tips, you can maintain your look longer and minimize your trips to the chair.

# THE GROOMING SOLUTION:

*Step One: Keep your back hairline neat.* One of the tell-tale signs of a required trim is the messy hairline on the back of your head, at the top of your neck. If you maintain this line on your own, you'll be able to put off the full deal for several weeks. Invest in a non-professional version of the electric clippers used by your hairstylist. Attach the length accessory and adjust it to the

> # REQUIRED GEAR
>
> • Electric trimmer with length attachment.
> • Hand mirror.
> • Mustache comb.
> • Mustache scissors (i.e., short and straight).

shortest setting. With your electric clippers in hand, stand in front of a wall mirror, grab a hand mirror, turn around and look at the back of your head. With the clipper in your most adept hand, run it over the hairline area. *Don't cut into your existing hairline.* Simply follow the line that you see. Trim your neckline once a week.

*Step Two: Keep the back of your neck clean.* Another haircut alarm? A hairy neck and back. To clean this up yourself, stand in front of a wall mirror, grab your hand mirror and turn around. Use your electric clippers to shave off the hair on your neck and back below the hairline you just cleaned up. Again, be careful not to alter the hairline itself. Trim accordingly every two to four weeks.

**Step Three: *Clean up those sideburns.*** Get yourself a good pair of mustache scissors (i.e., short, straight and sharp). Stand in front of a wall mirror with your shears in one hand and a small narrow-toothed mustache comb in the other. Comb each sideburn back towards your ears and then forward until you see the intended hairline of the sideburn and the scraggly pieces of hair that have grown long enough to mess up the line. With your scissors facing up towards your sideburn at a 45 degree angle, cut off these odd pieces using small choppy cuts. Target only one or two hairs per cut until you have cleaned up the entire sideburn. Trim your sideburns once a week.

# THE GROOMING ISSUE: USING HAIR JUNK

# THE FACTS:

Just as different hair types call for different washing routines (see the *Shampooing 101* section of this guidebook for more information), matching your hair type – oily, dry or damaged – with the right styling aids can make it easier to look your best.

# THE GROOMING SOLUTION:

*Oily hair.* Styling oily hair can be a challenge. Most styling products contain agents that, if applied in excess, will make your hair look even oilier. If you believe your hair is oily, avoid pomades, oily gels, styling creams and lotions. Opt for mousses, hair spray and "texturizing" products. Regardless of the styling products you choose, always use styling agents in moderation. Apply a dime-sized amount to your palm, rub your hands together and apply only half of the product in your hands to the ends of your hair. To avoid a greasy look, don't apply the product to your roots or scalp. If you find that you need more hair junk for your look, add small amounts in parts. After all, it's always easier to add product than to hop back into the shower and start over.

## REQUIRED GEAR

- Hair spray, mousses and "texturizing" lotion for *oily hair.*
- Gels, pomades, styling lotions and creams for *dry* or *damaged hair.*

*Dry or damaged hair.* SharpMen with dry or damaged hair should avoid mousses, hair sprays or gels not specifically designed for their hair type. Otherwise you'll find that the alcohol in these products will make your hair even more dry and hard to style. Opt for styling lotions, pomades, creams or "moisturizing" mousses. Apply a small quarter-sized amount of product to your palms, rub your hands together and apply at the ends of your hair – the driest areas that cause that "flyaway" look. Add small amounts of styling product as needed to avoid flaking.

*In-between hair.* If your hair is neither clearly oily nor dry, experiment with the products your hairstylist recommends. If you find that your hair flakes when you use gels, hair sprays or mousses, switch to light pomades, creams or lotions. Apply small amounts to the ends of your hair to avoid a greasy look.

**SHARPNOTE:** The sheer number of hair products on the market makes choosing a hairstyling aid confusing. To make matters worse, hair products seem to come in and out of "fashion." Should you care? Not really. Forget the fads and stick with what works for you.

# THE GROOMING ISSUE: COMBATING FRIZZY HAIR

## THE FACTS:

Whether curly or straight, some SharpMen's hair has a mind of its own. To avoid having your hair fly in all directions after a wash, consider using a hairstyling product made with *silica*. Silica is a plastic incorporated into styling products designed to control frizzy hair.

## THE GROOMING SOLUTION:

To use a silica-based product to control out-of-control frizz, apply a small amount to the palm of your hand, rub your palms together and apply small amounts to the ends, roots and some hair in between. Rather than applying to individual hairs, grab small "clumps" of hair when you apply. As with all products, start by using less than you think you need and add as you go.

## REQUIRED GEAR

• Silica-based hair product.

# THE GROOMING ISSUE:
## STRAIGHTENING CURLY LOCKS

# THE FACTS:

Curly hair is hard to fight. Think your hair is too curly for its own good? Has styling (read: controlling) your curly hair become a losing battle? Consider one of several processes for straightening curly hair.

# THE GROOMING SOLUTION:

**Blow-drying.** It is possible to "blow out" curly hair with a round brush and a blow-dryer. When you step out of the shower, towel dry your hair and apply a mousse or setting gel. Begin brushing out your hair with the round brush, holding and working the brush below the hair as you zap it with the blow-dryer. It takes patience, but your hair will eventually give in — until your next shower, that is.

**Chemical straightening.** If blowing out your hair isn't an option, consider having your hair chemically straightened. This is kind of like a reverse perm — the process *unwinds* hair instead of winding. Like any chemical process, chemical straightening must be done by a professional. If too much tension is placed on the hair while the straightening lotion is on, your hair could break off. If the lotion is left on too long, your hair could *dissolve*. In other words, don't try this at home.

When choosing a hairstylist to straighten your hair, ensure that he or she has experience with chemical straightening. Additionally, unless "bald" is your look, always request that your hairstylist use a "neutralizer" — key to protecting your hair during this harsh process.

**Chemical relaxing.** Alternatively, consider having your hair "relaxed" by a professional. The key to this process is *timing*. Once your hairstylist applies the relaxant, he or she must style your hair exactly the way you intend to wear it after the treatment. The hair will break down into this shape. Because this process requires precision, make a point of checking that the hairstylist you choose is experienced with relaxers and understands the hairstyle you have in mind *before* the treatment is applied.

And again, despite your buddies' "great" idea after a night of partying, *always* go to a professional. Cheapo over-the-counter products left on just a few minutes too long can cause hair to break and may leave you with bald patches.

**SHARPNOTE:** If you're trying to get "body" out of your chemical treatment, skip the perm. Consider using a thickening gel instead. Choose a product made with a lot of alcohol for maximum effect. Despite the fact that the alcohol is damaging to your hair, it will be a lot less damaging than a perm. Plus, the benefit of using hair junk over a permanent treatment is that you can wash it out when you're ready for a new look.

# THE GROOMING ISSUE: MAINTAINING LONG HAIR

## THE FACTS:

While easier on the wallet, long hair requires more maintenance than shorter styles. After all, you generally have to take better care of the stuff you want to keep for a longer period of time. What's more, neglected long hair shows it. If you find that your hair becomes more unruly and harder to style as it grows, your locks may be in need of some extra help.

### REQUIRED GEAR

• Shampoo.
• Conditioner.
• Detangling spray.
• Leave-in conditioning lotion.

## THE GROOMING SOLUTION:

To keep your long hair looking its best, take better care of the ends. When the ends become dry or are brushed too roughly, they tend to break and split (i.e., "split ends"). Why should you care? Because split ends cause your mane to thin and look, well, *ratty*.

*Step One: Condition.* To prevent this, consider using a conditioner after you shampoo. Apply the conditioner to the part of your hair that hangs below your ears all the way down to your ends. There's no need to use conditioner on your scalp and roots. Simply wipe off the excess conditioner from your hands onto this area. Let the product soak in for a few minutes while you soap up. Rinse your hair and towel dry.

*Step Two: Detangle.* Before laying into your hair with that chainsaw you call a hairbrush, spray on a detangling product. Detangling sprays prevent hair from snagging and breaking as you brush.

*Step Three: Brush and lube.* Begin by brushing out the ends and then work up to your scalp. Don't be rough; be patient. Follow with another "leave on" conditioning lotion, but only at the ends. This helps prevent that thrashed, "fly-away" look and makes your hair easier to style. Make a point of having your hair trimmed every two months or so to keep your ends from looking fried. If your long hair tends to get "frizzy," see the *Combating Frizzy Hair section* of this guidebook for more information.

# THE GROOMING ISSUE:
## DEALING WITH DANDRUFF

# THE FACTS:

Sure dandruff isn't the *worst* thing that could happen to a guy, but having white flakes sprinkling down your shoulders isn't exactly a great look.

Dandruff is actually a form of *eczema* that causes skin on your scalp to flake, but can also affect facial hair, chest hair, ears, and any area of the body where skin comes in contact with other skin (i.e., underarms, inner elbows, behind the knees and in the groin). Dandruff flaking can also cause itching and occasional redness.

> # REQUIRED GEAR
> • Dandruff shampoo or prescription treatment.

The cause of dandruff is unknown, although the tendency to develop it is hereditary. Dandruff can have both active and inactive periods; remaining invisible for months between flare-ups. It often affects SharpMen with oily skin and may leave skin looking greasy or unclean.

Because there is no known cure for dandruff, your best bet is to put your efforts towards *prevention*. Luckily, dandruff can be controlled by any number of relatively inexpensive and easy-to-use treatments.

# THE GROOMING SOLUTION:

**Over-the-counter shampoos.** Dandruff control can be as close as your local drugstore. These over-the-counter treatments differ from conventional shampoos in that they contain ingredients like *salicylic acid, coal tar, selenium sulfide, pyrithione zinc,* or *sulfur.* They may sound a bit fierce, but they're actually safe, gentle and appropriate for all hair types. When properly used, they greatly minimize dandruff flare-ups in all but the most severe cases.

While dandruff sufferers should shampoo daily, dandruff shampoos aren't designed to be used every day. Alternate your medicinal shampoo with your regular hair product, using your dandruff treatment every second or third washing.

If you find that one dandruff shampoo doesn't stop your flaking, consider picking up another product with a different active ingredient. Try several shampoos to determine which ingredient your scalp responds to best.

For facial hair dandruff, try lathering up with dandruff shampoo once a week. Allow the shampoo to soak in for five minutes before rinsing.

***Prescription lotions.*** Occasionally a case of dandruff will not respond to over-the-counter treatments. If you've tried several shampoos and haven't seen a decrease in flaking, see your doctor – preferably a dermatologist – who can examine your noggin and prescribe special scalp lotions. Prescription dandruff lotions often contain *selenium, corticosteroids* or *ketaconazole (Nizoral™)*, powerful ingredients that help control scalp flaking.

***Environmental controls.*** Dandruff can also become aggravated by a number of outside factors. In some cases, dry scalp skin and dandruff are related to stress, fatigue, infrequent shampooing, hair products containing alcohol (check out the ingredient list on your gel), tight-fitting or non-breathable hats and failing to dry hair and skin completely after showering. In the case of these aggravators, a few simple lifestyle changes can make a big difference.

Another tip? Participating in outdoor activities during warm weather also seems to reduce dandruff outbreaks. So *play ball*!

***SharpThreads for dandruff.*** Got dandruff? To minimize the evidence of your outbreak, consider wearing light colors. Lighter colors, especially white, can be somewhat effective in camouflaging dandruff flakes, whereas dark colors call attention to the winter wonderland on your shoulders.

**SHARPNOTE ONE:** It is common for dandruff shampoos to become less effective over time. If your shampoo of choice has lost its juice, simply switch to another one, and switch again when your second choice peters out.

**SHARPNOTE TWO:** While uncommon, some SharpMen's skin may become sensitive to one or more of the ingredients found in medicinal shampoos. If your skin becomes red after using one of these treatments, immediately discontinue use and consult your physician.

# THE GROOMING ISSUE: DATE & INTERVIEW HAIR

## THE FACTS:

Can a "good hair day" make a difference for a big interview or date? Studies indicate that to the extent a great hair day makes you feel more attractive, it will also make you feel more confident and positively affect your interactions with others. Hoping to project your best despite the nerves? In addition to practicing your smooth moves, take a moment to get that quaff under control.

## THE GROOMING SOLUTION:

*Step One: Schedule a haircut.* Instruct your hairstylist to take off less, rather than more. Prudence will avoid a last-minute disaster.

*Step Two: Invest* in a few of those hair-care products your hairstylist keeps trying to push off on you. Then spend a few more minutes having him or her teach you exactly how to apply and blow-dry for game day. Don't be shy – it's *your cash.* Don't leave until you feel confident that you have a solid understanding of how to re-create the look yourself.

*Step Three: Practice.* In the days before the event, make a habit of taking time to practice the routine. Like baseball or that musical instrument your mother always wanted you to play, you'll never get good unless you work the steps.

*Step Four: Allow for prep time.* Make a point of waking up earlier on the day of the date or interview, and leave yourself a nice cushion of time in which to redo your "do" as needed.

# THE GROOMING ISSUE:
## SHARP HANDS & FINGERNAIL CARE

# THE FACTS:

Sorry, buddy: girls *do* notice your hands. And while the rugged look is considered attractive, the beauty of dirty fingernails seems to be lost on the women-folk – especially while on dates with you.

Then there's the rough hand issue. Sure calluses are a man's way of proving his gender, but touching a girl's skin with those sandpaper-covered numbers is another complaint department altogether.

## REQUIRED GEAR

- Light moisturizing hand cream.
- Nail clippers or scissors.

With a few simple tips, it *is* possible to strike a balance between maintaining your guy-style hands and a hand shake that doesn't leave a scar.

# THE GROOMING SOLUTION:

*Hand cleaning for nails.* The best thing you can do for your nails is to keep your *hands* clean. Make a point of washing your hands after school and after dirt-magnet activities. Work your forefinger and thumbnails under the opposing nails to pick out dirt.

*Hand lube.* A little too into that hand-washing routine? You may find that frequent hand washing – particularly if you use harsh "antibacterial" soaps – can cause your hands and fingernails to become dry and scaly. To avoid this, get yourself a light moisturizing hand cream, available at your local drugstore or in your mom's medicine cabinet.

*Nail trimming.* Another easy way to keep hands and nails looking clean and attractive to the opposite sex is to simply trim your nails more often than you currently do. Keeping your nails short will prevent pockets of dirt from accumulating under your nails. For trimming, avoid using the clippers you use on your toes. Toenail clippers tend to break nails, leaving you with jagged nail pieces. Since you *clearly* don't intend to *file* down those nubs of yours, use the right tool for the job. Consider investing in a pair of scissors or clippers made especially for trimming fingernails.

***Cuticle patrol.*** Once you've trimmed your nails, take a moment to push back your cuticles — you know, those crusty boundaries of skin at the base of your nails. As your nails grow, the cuticle skin builds up and may develop a big "hump" of dead skin. After a while it may tear and bleed. Simply pushing these guys back before the geyser of blood erupts can make a big difference in how your nails look to others. To push back cuticles, simply use your opposing thumbnail to gently plow back the pieces of skin still hanging onto your nail. It's best to do this once a week or so, after you shower, when your skin is most pliable. As with anything, resist the urge to be too aggressive, or bacteria will take up residence at the base of your nail.

# THE GROOMING ISSUE: Fingernail Biters

## THE FACTS:

In this germ-conscious world, no one wants to shake hands with a guy who's just pulled his fingers out of his mouth. Despite this, fingernail-biting is surprisingly common among SharpMen. It's an easy habit to form but a tough one to stop. For many guys, nail-biting is so well-established that they barely realize how often they do it.

If you're ready to kick the habit, it's helpful to isolate your reasons for biting your nails in the first place:

### REQUIRED GEAR

- Nail clippers.
- Bad-tasting formula.
- Stress ball or pad of paper
- Gum or mints.

*Old habit.* Many young SharpMen can trace their nail-chomping back to when they were shy, self-conscious kids. Now they do it without thinking.

*Stress.* Tension is one of the leading reasons people begin – and continue – to bite their nails. Biting and picking become automatic reactions to the stress of an upcoming test, an important game or a worrisome problem.

*Habit triggered by another activity.* Often nail-biting is associated with an activity such as talking on the phone or watching television. Some guys bite their nails when bored or unoccupied (e.g., sitting on the bus or in class).

## THE GROOMING SOLUTION:

By isolating your reasons for biting your nails – and then briefly monitoring yourself under the same conditions – you'll be more likely to stop your hands from automatically going to your mouth. If willpower isn't enough, consider the following remedies:

*Put a formula on your nails.* Visit your local drugstore for one of several foul-tasting formulas designed to make your nails taste bad enough to turn you off of biting them – or at least alert you to when you do it unconsciously. Apply the colorless product to your fingernails and make a point of reapplying regularly to ensure that the foul taste remains strong.

***Keep your hands busy.*** Idle hands are likely to fuel your habit, so keep them busy. If you've found that you bite your nails when you are on the telephone, keep a pad of paper and pen handy for doodling. If you bite your nails when you're tense, consider adding a "stress ball" to your collection of stuff. The key is to do anything that keeps your hands busy and out of your mouth.

***Chew gum or mints.*** Seasoned nail-biters know that nail pieces and chewing gum are a bad combo. The next time you catch yourself chomping on your own body parts, pop a stick of gum or mint into your mouth.

***Use nail clippers.*** Always tempted to bite off a sharp nail edge or "even out" a nail that is a little longer than the others? Avoid these excuses by trimming your nails regularly and keeping a pair of nail clippers in your locker or gym bag.

***Make nail care a priority.*** Now that you've stopped biting your nails, take a few minutes to learn how to take care of them. See the *Sharp Hand and Fingernail Care* section of this guidebook for more information. By spending a bit of effort to get your hands in handshake-ready form, you'll be less likely to "fall off the wagon" and return to nail-biting.

# THE GROOMING ISSUE: UGLY FEET

## THE FACTS:

Ever go to the beach or wear sandals? Ugly feet can distract girls from your better attributes.

## THE GROOMING SOLUTION:

To solve the majority of unsightly foot problems, consider adding the following to your weekly grooming regimen:

**Wash** feet daily in *warm*, soapy water. Never soak your feet for more than ten minutes. Over-soaking can weaken the nails, which leads to breaking and chipping and, well, *ugly feet.*

**Dry feet** thoroughly after every wash, especially between the toes where smelly fungus feels most comfortable growing and your skin tends to become dry and cracked.

### REQUIRED GEAR

• Moisturizing lotion.
• Fresh socks for every day between laundry days.
• An alternate pair of canvas or leather shoes that fit well.

**Lube feet.** If the skin on your feet is dry and scaly, apply a moisturizing product. To prevent fungal growth, avoid applying moisturizer between your toes.

**Wear shoes that fit.** Tight-fitting shoes can contribute to the development of ingrown toenails – major players in the ugly feet phenomenon. For more information on preventing this condition, see the *Toenail Care & Ingrown Toenails* section of this guidebook.

**Change socks and wear shoes that breathe.** Change socks daily to avoid smelly, ugly fungal growth. When choosing your "everyday" shoes, opt for breathable, natural materials, such as canvas or leather. This is particularly important if your feet are prone to sweating. Alternate your "everyday" shoes every couple of days to ensure that they dry out completely. See the *Combating Athlete's Foot* section of this guidebook for more information.

# THE GROOMING ISSUE:
## TOENAIL CARE & INGROWN TOENAILS

## THE FACTS:

Even if you're not a sandals kind of guy, keeping your toenails trimmed properly will prevent ingrown toenails, a condition where poorly trimmed nails grow into the skin. Ingrown toenails are painful. They inhibit your ability to walk and wear shoes comfortably. Once they develop, the condition is best treated by a podiatrist, a doctor specializing in the care of feet. Simply trimming your toenails properly can prevent this painful foot ailment.

### REQUIRED GEAR

• Toenail clippers.
• Shoes that do not pinch at the toes.

## THE GROOMING SOLUTION:

The most important part of toenail care is simple: use clippers made for *toes*. Because fingernail clippers are not wide enough to cut straight across the toe, they force you to round out toenails as you trim – a big mistake. Improper cutting is a major cause of ingrown toenails.

On the other hand, clippers designed for use on toenails are wide enough to trim your toenail in one stroke – straight across – leaving the edges of your toenails above the skin on either side. When trimming, make a point of cutting straight from end to end, as rounding out the sides will make it more likely that your shoes will push your skin over the toenail and cause the sides of the nail to grow into your skin. *Ouch.* The best news? Toenail clippers are cheap; another good reason to get the right tool for the job.

Purchasing shoes that fit properly is another easy way to avoid ingrown toenails. Pass on any shoe that pinches at the toes.

# THE GROOMING ISSUE:
## COMBATING ATHLETE'S FOOT

# THE FACTS:

Ever have an itch on your foot that makes you want to shove your leg into the freezer? Ever try it? Before compromising the ecosystems of major household appliances, check out the facts about athlete's foot and what you can do to get it under control.

Athlete's foot is caused by a fungus that grows in moist, warm areas. The condition is generally associated with peeling skin or areas of redness on the feet. Some guys also suffer from uncontrollable itching and *really* bad foot odor. The bottom line? If you have this condition, your feet look and smell *bad*.

## REQUIRED GEAR

- Shoetrees.
- Fresh socks for every day between laundry days.
- An alternate pair of canvas or leather shoes that fit well.
- Pool or shower shoes.
- Foot powder or spray.

# THE GROOMING SOLUTION:

The best way to control athlete's foot is to avoid the circumstances under which it develops.

*Change.* A chief cause of athlete's foot is remnant moisture in the inner leather lining of your shoes. That's right; sometimes the fungus develops *in your shoes.* Make a point of changing shoes as often as practical, giving each pair a chance to dry.

*Choose.* If your feet spend the majority of their days in shoes, choose shoes made of leather or canvas – materials that allow feet to breathe.

*Air dry.* When you take off your shoes, don't stuff your socks back into them - this prevents your shoes from airing out properly and creates a nice, moist environment for the growth of fungus. Instead, place your shoes in a well-ventilated area between use:

> • *For leather shoes and boots*, purchase and use cedar shoetrees. Quality shoetrees help absorb moisture and sustain the shape

of your leather shoes and boots.
- *For athletic shoes,* loosen the shoelaces and pull the tongues out, thereby exposing the interior to light and air.

*Change again.*  Avoid wearing the same socks two days in a row. If you have a chance to do so, switch to a dry pair of socks after school and after the gym or a game.

*Sprinkle or spray.*  If your feet are prone to sweating, visit your drugstore for foot powder or foot powder spray.  Sprinkle or spray the powder on your feet and into your socks to cut down on the moisture caused by sweating.

*Wash.* When you wash your feet, make a point of cleaning between the toes with soap and water. Then thoroughly dry your feet, particularly in between your toes.

*Wear sandals or flip-flops* in locker rooms at the gym and around the pool to protect your feet from other guys' fungi. That's right; *the fungus you carry may not be your own...*

If you suspect that you've developed athlete's foot, see a podiatrist who can prescribe anti-fungal medication to control the fungus and the itching.  In extreme circumstances, your doctor may recommend nail surgery.

# THE GROOMING ISSUE: DRY, CRACKED HEELS

## THE FACTS:

Dry, cracked heels are a big problem for lots of guys. Unlike girls, many young SharpMen are less likely to moisturize when they get out of the shower. In winter or during seasons when bare feet and open-toe shoes are in and out of water, the skin on the bottom of your feet can

### REQUIRED GEAR

• Gentle, non-drying soap.
• Antibacterial ointment.
• Petroleum jelly.
• Gym socks.

dry out. The result? A painful cracking of the skin on the bottoms of your feet and possible infection.

## THE GROOMING SOLUTION:

The following tips will help soothe and heal dry, cracked heels:

*Step One: Clean.* Your first job is to ensure that the cracked areas of your skin – basically exposed wounds – do not become infected. Wash your feet thoroughly before you turn in at night. Use a gentle soap less likely to further irritate your skin.

*Step Two: Disinfect.* Apply an over-the-counter antibacterial ointment to the cracked areas. Use a lot.

*Step Three: Lube up.* After applying the ointment, take half of a golf ball-sized amount of a petroleum jelly, and slather it all over your feet – particularly on the area where your heels are cracked.

*Step Four: Cover up.* Once your feet are well-lubed, slowly put a gym sock over each foot, being careful not to wipe off too much of the jelly and ointment.

*Step Five: Go to sleep.* In the morning, remove the gym socks and wipe off any excess jelly that did not absorb. If possible, remain bare-foot for a while to give the open wounds time to dry out.

**Step Six: Reapply.** When you get out of the shower, take a *small* amount of petroleum jelly and rub it on the dry part of your heel before putting on your shoes. Wash, dry and repeat this small application when you get home from school, but this time leave your shoes off to let your heels breathe.

**Step Seven: Repeat** the sock routine for about a week or until your heels start looking better. You may want to do this more often during winter and other drying times of the year.

**Step Eight: Keep an eye on things.** If you notice your cracked heels getting worse or looking red and inflamed, see a physician. You may be allergic to one of the products used. Your doctor will check for infection and give you something for your heels that does not contain the chemical agent you are reacting to.

# THE GROOMING ISSUE: CORNS & CALLUSES

## THE FACTS:

Guys who do a lot of walking or engage in athletic activities often have feet riddled with corns and calluses – great for walking on glass, bad for your feet.

> ### REQUIRED GEAR
>
> - Shoes that fit the shape of your foot.
> - Thongs or sandals.
> - Corn or callus remover.

Corns and calluses are caused by a thickening of the skin, which builds up in layers on the toes (corns) and heels (calluses) of your feet. This build-up can cause shoes and boots to pinch and become less comfortable.

## THE GROOMING SOLUTION:

If you're self-conscious about the build-up of skin on your feet, consider:

**Your shoes.** Like blisters, corns and calluses are often caused by ill-fitting shoes that rub against the skin on your feet. Make a point of choosing shoes and boots that fit the shape of your foot – regardless of what everyone else is wearing.

**Your habits.** Walking barefoot is another cause of corns and calluses. Consider throwing on a pair of thongs or sandals the next time you're planning a stroll.

**Removal.** If removal of corns and calluses is your plan, you'll find a variety of no-pain and no-brainer remedies sold over-the-counter at your local drugstore. Most require a one-time application.

**They're back.** If your corns and calluses persist, you may have a problem that cannot be remedied at home. For example, you may walk or position your foot in a way that promotes the growth of corns and calluses. Visit a podiatrist, a doctor specializing in foot care, for an "orthotic" insert, a device worn in your shoes that corrects foot position and abnormal foot motion.

# THE GROOMING ISSUE:
## IMPROVING YOUR POSTURE

# THE FACTS:

The most obvious drawback to poor posture is a slumped look that conveys a lack of confidence – to girls, to other guys, and anyone else who happens to see you. Internally there can be other, more serious problems. Standing, walking or sitting incorrectly can cause muscle tension, unnatural strain on ligaments and joints, improperly aligned bones, headaches, fatigue, shoulder, neck and back pain and other adverse effects on the position and function of your internal organs.

## REQUIRED GEAR

• Several small pillows.
• Back support cushion.

How's your posture? What looks fine to you may look like a "walking question mark" to others. To determine whether your posture could use some home improvement, ask a friend or doctor to watch the way you walk, sit and stand. Alternatively, study your reflection as you walk past a storefront. Are your shoulders slumped forward? Is your head down? Or do you hold your back stiff and your head thrown forward? If the answer is yes to any of these questions, your body – and your image – could benefit from a posture revamping.

# THE GROOMING SOLUTION:

*Sleep correctly.* Avoid sleeping on your stomach. Instead, aim to sleep on your back or on your side. If you prefer to sleep on your back, place a pillow under your head and shoulders, another rolled pillow or "neck roll" under your neck, and a third pillow under your knees. This position will provide maximum support to your spine. For SharpMen who sleep on their side, place a pillow under your head, making sure that your neck is supported and that your head is level with your spine. Place a second pillow between your bent knees. If you find that you tend to roll forward once you nod off, place a third pillow in front of your chest.

*Lift with your knees.*  When lifting objects, bend at the knees and use your leg and stomach muscles to lift, rather than your back. If you find that you can't help but lift with your back, consider getting a weight belt for the gym and other lifting activities.

*Carry close to your chest.*  When carrying heavy items, try to hold them close to your chest. This simple change will take some of the strain from your shoulders and back and help improve your posture.

*Stand with one foot raised.*  If you must stand for a sustained amount of time, place one foot on a chair or stool, changing feet often.  If you can't use a footstool, occasionally shift your weight between your feet, bending slightly at the knees and keeping your spine straight.

*Support your lower back while seated.*  When sitting for long periods of time (i.e., more than an hour and a half), place a rolled towel or cushion behind your lower back and push your rear into the back of the chair. Try to position your knees so that they are level with, or slightly above, your hips with your feet flat on the floor.

*Adjust your driving seat.*  If you drive, position your seat close enough to the wheel to avoid leaning in.  Position the headrest to support the middle of your head and sit with your back firmly against the seat.

*Walk straight.*  When walking, try to keep your head up and eyes straight ahead. Hold your shoulders back, but not to the point where the position requires you to tense up or push your head forward.

*Stretch regularly.* If you must sit for long periods of time, take a break and walk around every hour or so.  If strolling is not an option, try stretching in your seat.  For example, look up, raise your arms over your head, inhale deeply and hold this position for 10 seconds. Repeat six times. Alternatively, slowly roll your head clockwise three times and then counterclockwise three times.

*Get regular exercise and eat properly*. Overall good health always helps to maintain your body's top form. Activities like cycling or swimming are particularly beneficial for strengthening your back and improving your posture. Eating fresh fruits and vegetables, drinking eight glasses of water per day and recharging your body with regular sleep intervals will help fight fatigue and dehydration — two factors that contribute to poor posture.

# THE GROOMING ISSUE: REMOVING BACK HAIR

## THE FACTS:

Most young SharpMen don't have hairy backs – yet; others have enough hair to serve as a winter coat. The "right" look is a matter of personal preference. For those guys who prefer less back hair for summer activities, temporary and permanent hair removal options abound.

## THE GROOMING SOLUTION:

*Shaving.* Although shaving is by far your least expensive option, it is also the least permanent. Nonetheless, for guys who need a quick fix, shaving may be your best bet.

Will shaving body hair make it grow back thicker? No – that's a myth. Neither shaving, trimming or cutting head or body hair makes hair grow any faster or thicker. So go for it.

> ## REQUIRED GEAR
>
> *For shaving:*
> • Razor.
> • Light moisturizing balm.
> • Someone to shave you.

Regardless of whether you use an electric or traditional razor, one basic rule applies: *don't shave yourself.* Shaving a hard-to-reach area like your back can spell disaster. Not only will you miss large spots of hair, you'll be more likely to injure yourself in the process. Ask your folks or your buddy to help out.

Once you're set up, hop into the shower. The heat and water will open up your pores and soften your skin and back hairs, making it easier for you to shave and harder for you to cut yourself. Softening skin will also help prevent razor burn and other inflammations.

If you plan to use a traditional razor, ask your assistant to apply a thick layer of shaving cream to the designated shaving area. This is an easy way to control just how far up your shoulders and down your back your assistant will shave – *before* it's too late. Ask your helper to use short strokes down your back rather than shaving against the grain of hair growth. Remind him or her to rinse the razor in hot water every five strokes to prevent snags and cuts.

Once you're done shaving, finish off by applying a light moisturizer to prevent the razor burn and breakouts that often result from post-shave dryness and irritation.

*Waxing.* Another great short-term hair removal method is waxing. Unlike shaving, which only lasts about three days, most guys only need to wax their backs once a month.

Often used by athletes, waxing is performed in a private room at a salon or spa. The basic method goes like this: a licensed aesthetician (what used to be called a "beautician") warms a pot of wax and uses a large tongue depressor to spread the wax onto your back. He or she places a small piece of cloth onto the wax-covered area. The cloth and wax combination is then quickly removed – taking your hair and roots with it. Although this might seem painful – and it can be – the pain only lasts about thirty seconds, and is a small price to pay for hair-free skin.

One problem associated with waxing is the possibility of a post-wax acne breakout or rash. To prevent this, most attendants use a pre-wax treatment, like a powder. After the treatment, the aesthetician may apply alcohol to remove the wax and disinfect. Taking a shower directly after a waxing also helps reduce the possibility of breakouts and redness.

*Laser treatments.* Although not commonly used by young SharpMen, laser hair removal uses an invisible beam of light to permanently disable the growth of hair follicles. Of course, nothing is magic. The small laser-directing tip treats only dime-sized to one-inch areas per "shot." Consequently, you may require a few hours per treatment and several return visits to treat your entire back. Laser back hair removal can be uncomfortable and tends to be more expensive than other treatments.

*Electrolysis.* Also not commonly used by young SharpMen is electrolysis, a hair removal treatment that uses a small needle to pass electric currents to the root of the hair, thereby killing the root and permanently arresting the regrowth of your back hair – *one at a time.* The upside? You can remove your back hair forever. The downside? Like laser hair removal, electrolysis can be painful, expensive and may last up to a year, depending on the amount of hair on your back.

**SHARPNOTE:** Are you prone to back acne? If so, waxing can further irritate this sensitive condition. Consider waiting until your back clears up before using a waxing treatment to remove back hair. For more information, see the *Preventing Back Acne* section of this guidebook.

# THE GROOMING ISSUE: PREVENTING BACK ACNE

## THE FACTS:

Never get to play the "skins" team in B-ball? Always feel like all eyes are on your back in the locker room? Treat your back acne and both concerns will fade away.

## THE GROOMING SOLUTION:

*Choose right.* You may not realize it, but like other parts of your body, your back has *a lot* of oil glands. But unlike your face or, in some cases, your arms, your back is covered up all day. If you wear breathable cotton undershirts to keep sweat from staining your clothes, your cotton Ts may be contributing to your back acne.

### REQUIRED GEAR

- Loofah scrubber with a long handle.
- Acne medication.
- Non-absorbent undershirts.
- Oil-free sunscreen.

Because cotton is so absorbent, it holds sweat in the fabric – and close to your skin – all day. If you find that you have problems with back acne, consider switching to synthetic T-shirts that keep moisture away from your skin. Similarly, after workouts and other physical activities, change out of sweaty cotton gym clothes and uniforms as soon as practical.

*Change right.* Make a point of wearing a clean shirt or T-shirt every day – even if it's had time to "breathe" overnight, a shirt that has absorbed back skin oils is more likely to cause back acne.

*Wash right.* Ready to hit the shower? Visit your local drugstore for a long-handled "loofah" sponge or other abrasive scrubbing aid to remove dead skin cells while you soap up. Dead skin cells clog up pores and lead to breakouts. The more often you remove these dead skin cells the better off your back will be.

With your loofah in hand, lather up and scrub away. The idea is to *gently* remove excess cells; apply enough pressure to do the job, but not so much as to cause redness or skin irritation. For those SharpMen who feel that their backs need extra help, consider using a cleanser designed especially for body acne.

**Dry right.** Use a fresh towel to dry your back thoroughly. Covering open pores on a damp back is an invitation to acne and skin irritation.

**Treat right.** You can also spot treat your back acne with a topical gel or lotion. Keep in mind that, because back acne is cooped up in your sweaty clothes all day, it may be slower to respond than the blemishes on your face. For this reason, only apply the medication where you actually *have* acne. Otherwise, you'll end up drying out your back and creating red and itchy areas.

**Hairy considerations.** Do you have long head hair? If your mane hangs against your skin or creates a small sweat bath when it comes in contact with your T-shirt, your locks may be aggravating the pores on your back. Consider washing your hair more often to prevent oil build-up, giving it a trim or wearing it up and away from your back.

**Sun treatments.** Many SharpMen who suffer from winter back break-outs look forward to summer – when baring their back to the sun seems to temporarily clear up their acne problem. But beware: beyond the increased risk of skin cancer, blasts of sun exposure may clear up your back at the expense of scarring sensitive zit-covered skin. Then, come winter, your back may look worse than ever.

Use sunscreen when exposing your back – or any other part of our skin – to the sun. Worried that goopy sunscreen will promote more breakouts? Pick up an oil-free sunscreen that protects your skin from sun, scarring and zits. For more information, see the *Safe Tanning* section of this guidebook.

**SHARPNOTE:** Most over-the-counter acne medications contain *ben-zoyl peroxide*. This effective acne-fighting ingredient may bleach your clothing if you don't allow the medication to fully absorb and dry prior to putting on your clothes.

# THE GROOMING ISSUE: MOLES & SKIN TAGS

# THE FACTS:

In a world where clear skin is hip, many young SharpMen feel that that their moles and skin tags are not. And while these skin marks are normal, they demand some attention and care.

Moles and skin tags are non-malignant (non-cancerous) skin growths that tend to be inherited. Almost everyone has a few moles; most people have between ten and forty throughout their body. They usually appear in childhood or adolescence and continue to develop into a SharpMan's forties. Moles can be small or large; flesh-colored, yellow-brown, or black; flat or raised; smooth, hairy or wart-like. Many moles begin as small, flat spots and slowly become raised and grow larger in diameter. The majority are round or oval, no bigger than a pencil eraser. Over many years, moles may flatten again, become flesh-colored, or even disappear.

In the same family of moles are skin tags; soft, small, flesh-colored or other-colored growths, usually occurring in multiples on the neck, eyelids, armpits and groin. Skin tags are generally harmless but may be irritating, especially if they catch on clothing or rub against your collar.

Years ago, studies erroneously linked skin tags with colon cancer. Since then, researchers have found that simply gaining weight can increase the development of skin tags.

# THE GROOMING SOLUTION:

*Care for moles and skin tags.* While most are harmless, some moles can cause considerable health problems. For this reason it is necessary to properly care for and monitor your moles. For example:

- Moles that suddenly change in color or size should be evaluated by a physician to ensure that the change does not indicate *melanoma*, a serious form of skin cancer. Other warning signs include itching, crusting, pain and bleeding.
- Exposing moles to the sun increases the usual risk of skin cancer. Keep your moles covered and out of the sun.

- Don't pick at your moles. If a mole is irritating you, speak to your doctor about having it removed.
- By contrast, skin tags are fairly harmless, rarely "changing" into something that requires medical attention or treatment.

**Removal of moles.** While the majority of moles do not *require* removal, they are often removed for cosmetic reasons. Your physician can remove moles by excision, liquid nitrogen, or banding, although most people choose to have their moles removed by a plastic surgeon or dermatologist to minimize scarring.

Moles that have developed on the surface of the skin can also be shaved off by a doctor in a "shave biopsy." The area around the mole is numbed with local anesthesia and the mole is shaved off. This procedure does not generally produce scarring, however, in some cases a whitish discoloration remains.

Moles that grow deeper, into the second layer of the skin, require a "punch biopsy," wherein local anesthesia is applied and a small, cookie cutter-like device is used to remove the mole. As a precautionary measure, each mole removed is sent to a laboratory to ensure that it's non-cancerous.

**Removal of skin tags.** By contrast, removal of skin tags is less involved and is often performed by a general physician. Methods include freezing the tag with liquid nitrogen, tying off the tag with a thread or suture to cut off the blood supply, or cutting off the tag with a scalpel or scissors – all with minimal patient discomfort.

# THE GROOMING ISSUE: SAFE TANNING

## THE FACTS:

Sure you don't *want* skin cancer when you're older, but is the price of healthy skin a blinding white torso? Not at all. Rather than spending time and money on a trip to the sunny side of the street, many SharpMen are discovering a

> ### REQUIRED GEAR
>
> • Tanning cream, spray or accelerator.
> • Sunscreen SPF 15 or higher.

faster, safer and less expensive option: *self-tanning products* – grooming aids that safely change the color of your skin from white to golden.

In the past, tanning creams were tricky: most turned skin orange, rather than golden brown, and if not applied evenly, they produced a "splotchy" effect. Today's re-engineered, easier-to-use products have given tanning creams a better name.

## THE GROOMING SOLUTION:

If you'd like to use a tanning cream or spray, consider the following tips for best results:

*Clean.* Begin with clean, dry skin.

*Apply* a light coat of the cream or spray on your skin. Use less than you think you need.

*Blend* the cream or spray quickly and evenly on your skin.

When applying to the face, first apply the product to your hands, rub your hands together to spread the product and then blend evenly onto the face. Avoid direct contact with the eye area; the skin around the eyes is generally lighter in color than other facial skin, so this will actually look more natural.

*Stop.* You may not notice an immediate color change after your initial application, but resist the temptation to apply more. Your new color will become obvious in two to four hours.

**Wash** hands in hot soapy water immediately after using the product.

**Wait** to put on your clothing until the tanning lotion has dried completely. Avoid swimming and bathing for an hour after your application.

By giving yourself a nice "base" coat of color, you'll be less self-conscious about hitting the water and less likely to fry your skin. If you'd like to slowly transition your faux color to a safe tan, generously apply sunscreen whenever you expose your skin to the sun and your color-from-a-bottle will slowly transition into a long-lasting summer tan.

# THE GROOMING ISSUE: TATTOO REMOVAL

# THE FACTS:

Many young SharpMen look at their arms and wonder, "What was I thinking? I don't even know this girl anymore..." For those who want to erase what they can't - or prefer not to - remember, professional tattoo removal may be the answer.

In the past, techniques for removing tattoos were pretty harsh. Whether *dermabrasion, salabrasion, Argon* or *CO2* lasers were used, red, blue and black ink could not be removed successfully, and the patient was often left with unsightly scar tissue. Today, new laser treatments yield much better results with red, blue and black inks and significantly reduce the formation of scar tissue. Treatments are usually administered by dermatologists and other physicians certified in laser treatment.

# THE GROOMING SOLUTION:

*Sun power.* Just as excessive sun exposure can fade and dilute tattoo lines over time, the new types of tattoo removal treatments use the energy of light to break down and fade tattoo ink. The advantage is that new tattoo removal lasers do this much more quickly and safely. The lasers are designed to channel only one or two specific wavelengths of light in very short, powerful bursts, thereby breaking down tattoo inks and causing minimal damage to the skin, as compared to sun exposure or other tattoo removal methods. The wavelengths pass through the skin and break down tattoo ink so that it can be filtered out by the patient's body.

*Success rates.* It's hard for any procedure to work for all tattoos. Why? Over one hundred types of ink are used all over the world – none regulated by governmental agencies. More mysterious are the amounts and skin depths at which the inks are administered by various tattoo artists. For this reason, it is nearly impossible for physicians to predict how well a tattoo will fade before treatment. In most cases about ninety-five percent of the tattoo fades. Blue, black and red inks fade best; orange and purples next best; while green and yellow inks are the most difficult colors to remove.

***Pain considerations.*** New treatments also make tattoo removal a lot less painful. The lasers used emit "pulses," or short bursts of light, that are felt for less than a second at a time. The feeling has been compared to a very short snap of a rubber band or a small amount of hot bacon grease on your arm – *but only for a second.* Only very sensitive SharpMen will require anesthesia, and then only locally.

After treatment, some SharpMen may experience pinpoint-sized bleeding in the immediate removal area, which will be cleaned and bandaged. You'll be able to shower the following day so long as you don't scrub the wound.

***Treatment time.*** Does one shot do it? Not exactly. Removal of professional tattoos requires about five or six treatments, while amateur tattoos only require three or four sessions each spaced about a month apart. The number of sessions required depends on the amount and types of inks used and how deep they lie beneath the skin. Only the "worst" cases require ten visits or more.

# THE GROOMING ISSUE: Using Cologne Without Going Overboard

# THE FACTS:

You want to smell good, but no guy should smell *too* good.

Despite what cologne manufacturers would like you to believe, the best cologne application is a subtle one. Think of cologne in two ways: one, as insurance in case you reek; and two, as a special signature for those who come close enough to notice. In both cases, there's no need to go overboard. Just think *subtlety*, and your message will be just as strong.

# THE GROOMING SOLUTION:

To manage your cologne application, consider the following:

***Choose your tools.*** For those young SharpMen who have a hard time regulating the amount of cologne they apply, stick with a spray product. Never exceed two pumps of the spray. If it is not possible to get a spray in your fragrance of choice, do what you can to avoid "splashing" like the actors in those aftershave commercials. After all, once the dam is open, volume can get out of control faster than you think.

***Pick your application point.*** Certain areas of the body have a higher "burn rate" than others. These hot spots, frequently used by women, include the inner wrist, neck and other areas exposed to air. To keep these areas reeking all day, you'll have to start with a lot of scent in the morning – which often means that you arrive to school stinking like *Pepe Le Pew*. We don't recommend this.

Instead, apply a small amount to your hands and rub the cologne (or simply spray) to your *chest, back, thighs* or any other part of your body that is not exposed to air. This allows the scent of your cologne to emanate slowly and relatively evenly throughout the day.

**SHARPNOTE:** While it may be tempting, don't get carried away by the intimate possibilities of cologne. Avoid applying fragrance to your, uh, *organs*, or you'll be suffering from potentially painful consequences for a while.

# THE GROOMING ISSUE: Choosing Cologne

## THE FACTS:

Tempted to save time and splash on any old scent you've gotten from family and friends? Keep in mind that fragrances come in different concentration levels and scent families that are appropriate for various occasions and lifestyles. Sound complicated? Picking your signature scent is easier than you might think once you understand the basics.

## THE GROOMING SOLUTION:

*Choosing a concentration level.* Fragrances come in varying levels of concentration, meaning some are stronger than others. For example, aftershave has the least amount of fragrance, *eau de toilette* has more, and *eau de cologne* contains even more. (*Eau de parfum* actually has the most, but this concentration is generally reserved for women's fragrances.) The higher the level of concentration you choose, the less cologne is required for a strong application.

*Choosing a scent.* Like descriptions of wine, a discussion of cologne scent characteristics can sound more like a botany lesson than an easy-to-understand guide to choosing a fragrance you like. To keep things simple, the following scents are divided into four categories: casual-daytime wear, power wear, evening wear, and date wear:

*Casual-daytime wear* fragrances tend to be light, clean, crisp, and citrusy, and are appropriate for school days, weekends and casual outings. Look for scents that combine rosemary, lime, mandarin, iris, vanilla, musk, and cedar or mint, lavender, sandalwood, cedar and amber.

*Power wear* fragrances are generally refreshing, sharp and spicy and give off a "commanding" aura that is appropriate for days when you have a class presentation or a big interview — when used in *moderation*. Look for fragrances that blend small amounts patchouli and sandalwood with woodsy undertones.

*Evening wear.* For young SharpMen who want to get the crowd's attention as they enter that big party, evening wear colognes are strong, exotic and refined. Look for fragrances that blend oak musk, lavender, grapefruit, and mandarin, lemon, orange, lavender, sage, cedar and believe it or not, tobacco.

*Date scents* are generally heavier and spicier, designed for more intimate occasions. Look for blends of cloves, jasmine, rose, coriander, vanilla, honey and even grass, or lemons, oranges and bergamot, combined with deeper notes of clove, coriander, nutmeg and aromatic wood. Studies indicate that the "right" scents can make people feel more romantically inclined.

**Buying a scent.** Ready to put your cash on the barrel? Take a small bag of coffee beans to your local department store and sniff around. Ask the salesperson to recommend scents that combine those ingredients that meet your fragrance needs (see above).

Ask for and spray the testers on small pieces of cardboard rather than your arms. Between each sniff, breathe into the coffee bean bag to "clean" your smell palette. Now try another. When you've narrowed your choices down to two or three, spray a small amount on different parts of your arms, make note of what you sprayed where and then walk away from the counter.

After about an hour, smell your skin again to see which scent you prefer. You'll find that the oils and the individual chemistry of your skin will change the way each cologne smells on you. Make your selection based on these "mature" scents.

# THE GROOMING ISSUE: MAKING YOUR COLOGNE LAST

## THE FACTS:

Maintaining a stockpile of cologne can be expensive. Of course, the longer you make it last, the less you will have to spend.

## THE GROOMING SOLUTION:

To get more mileage out of your cologne, consider the following:

***Skin type.*** The length of time your cologne lasts is affected by your skin type. If you have oily skin, you're in luck: scent will last longer on you due to your skin's higher moisture content – potentially up to five or six hours. As such, go ahead and ease up on your applications.

Young SharpMen with dry skin will find that their colognes don't have quite as much stamina. Rather than applying more in the morning, consider dividing your morning routine by reapplying smaller amounts between activities.

***Quality versus price.*** While low-cost knock-offs of popular colognes abound, the higher-quality ingredients and essential oils found in the real thing are likely to last several *hours* longer per application. Sure, you'll save a few bucks on the front end, but you'll also find yourself reapplying more often and depleting your supply much more quickly. Not much of a deal.

**SHARPNOTE:** Because cologne generally lasts only four to six hours, consider keeping an extra bottle in your gym bag or locker for a quick reapplication before you head out for an after-school activity. Many types of cologne also come in trial and travel sizes perfect for this purpose. Of course, always remember that scents begin emanating the second you open the bottle. To avoid becoming the joke of your school (think "Tulip Boy"), remove yourself (and your bottle) to the men's room before uncorking and reapplying.

# THE GROOMING ISSUE: Storing Cologne

# THE FACTS:

Again, cologne is expensive. By simply using and storing it properly, you'll have to buy it less often. In fact, with proper storage and usage, high-quality cologne can last between five and seven years.

# THE GROOMING SOLUTION:

To maximize the life of your cologne, consider the following:

*Packaging.* Colognes release their scent the moment you uncork them. The less often they are opened, the more powerful your fragrance will remain. Similarly, contaminants found on all hands — even freshly showered ones — weaken the scent of cologne. As such, spray colognes tend to last longer than splash colognes — you use less with every application and the fragrance does not come into contact your hands or the outside air due to the spray applicator.

*Storage.* According to fragrance experts, cologne should be stored in a manner similar to wine. Should you ask your folks to start building that cologne cellar in the basement? Not necessarily. Simply avoid exposing your colognes to heat, sunlight, and air. A bathroom cabinet or counter is fine, so long as the counter isn't exposed to direct sunlight. If possible, store the fragrance in its original box if you plan to wait awhile before using it.

# THE GROOMING ISSUE:

## SHARPGROOMING IN THE LOCKER ROOM

## THE FACTS:

Due to heat in the showers and steam room and the ever-present sweat and other bodily fluids, your school locker room or local gym become a haven for the growth of bacteria and germs. Do you walk around barefoot? If you do, you'll be a prime candidate for athlete's foot. Do you sit in the steam room and rest your back against the wall? If the guy before you had a skin rash, your chances of contracting it rise. Similarly, if the guy who shaved in the sink before you cut himself and failed to rinse the faucet, using the sink exposes you to infection. *Eeeeew.*

### REQUIRED GEAR

• Shower shoes or thongs.
• Clean towel.
• Clean socks.
• Toiletry kit.

## THE GROOMING SOLUTION:

*Relax.* Arming yourself against the unseen hazards of the locker room is as simple as following a few tips:

*Cover your feet.* Wear flip flops, sandals or water shoes. In addition to preventing slips and spills, simply wearing something to protect your feet provides a line of defense against other guys' athlete's foot and other infections you could do without.

*Wash your towels.* Some schools and gyms provide clean towels. For those that require you to bring your own, make it a clean one. Don't let the same damp towel sit in your locker or gym bag week after week. Damp towels can quickly become breeding grounds for bacteria and germs, especially after you've hung them on the rack while shower-ing – where other guys' sweaty towels were before. Ever seen a janitor wiping down towel racks between customers? Neither have we. Make a point of swapping out your towels every few days.

*Wear a towel or swim trunks while steaming.* While the guy next to you may hit the sauna, steam room or hot tub in the buff, doctors rec-ommend wearing swim trunks or sitting on and wrapping your lower body in a towel. This simply act of modesty protects you from pubic lice and any bacteria present on the steam room seat. Wanna lean back against the tile? Consider putting a towel between the open pores on your back and the last guy who got cozy in the steam.

***Change your socks***. Bring a clean pair of socks to change into after your workout. Wearing the same pair of sweaty socks (particularly if they've picked up bacteria off the floor of the locker room) promotes the growth of athlete's foot.

***Dry your back.*** A young SharpMan's back is one of the hardest parts of the body to keep clean — and therefore the most vulnerable. Drying it thoroughly will help prevent the development of back acne and help protect you from the spread of bacteria you may have picked up by leaning against the walls of steam rooms, tanning beds, saunas or hot tubs.

***Separate toiletries.*** Always keep your toothbrush, soap and razor in a separate bag or container from the rest of your workout gear to avoid spreading bacteria from your clothing and towel to your toothbrush bristles and other grooming products. A toiletry bag will protect these items in addition to providing an alternative surface for resting your grooming gear on while at the sink. Regardless of what you do at home, realize that setting toothbrushes and razors on locker room sinks is *not* a great idea.

***Wash right.*** If you don't intend to shower at the gym, wash your hands before heading out. The build-up of bacteria and germs is common on workout equipment and machinery — especially during cold season.

# THE GROOMING ISSUE:
## THE TWO-MINUTE SAFETY CHECK

# THE FACTS:

Most young SharpMen would be surprised to learn what details they fail to notice before running out the door. Of course, these are the very details that are noticed (and snickered at) by your friends, arch-enemies and the ladies you were hoping to impress. *Oops.*

# THE GROOMING SOLUTION:

The next time you head out the door, take two minutes for this no-brainer safety check:

*Step One: Head.* Starting at the top, check your hair; it is neat? If possible, keep your hair trimmed, including the stuff on the back of your neck that makes you look like a primate between trips to the barber. See the *Making Your Haircut Last* section of this guidebook for more information.

Check your eyes: is there gunk in the corners? Dig it out. Wash your glasses; spots on the lenses can be distracting to the girls you approach.

Look up your nostrils; not the greatest view, but it's better for you to check then for someone *else* to see it, not tell you about it and let you walk around with it all day (or at least until it falls off onto your shirt).

*Ears:* get out the cotton swabs. Gently clean the outer canal. Resist the urge to jam the swab into your ear and mess up your eardrums. See the *Ear Care* section of this guidebook for more information.

*Cheeks and chin:* any shaving nicks or food crumbs?

*Step Two: Body.* Did you remember to use deodorant? Take a quick look at the back of your shirt; is the collar right and the tag tucked in? How about the rest of your clothing – on a scale of one to ten, how clean or wrinkle-free does it look? Got a pet? Could you use a quick sweep with a lint brush?

**Step Three: Hands and Feet.** How gross do you fingernails look? Could they use a trim? How about dirt under the nails – if you can see it, it *will* gross out the ladies. See the *Hands & Fingernail Care* section of this guidebook for more information.

Now take a quick look at your shoes; could they use a quick towel dusting? How about your shoe laces – are they torn or ratty? Could they use a replacement?

**Try the Two-Minute Safety Check**. A quick sweep before school, dates and even before dreaded trips to see your relatives can go a long way towards maintaining your sharp look. You'll be surprised by what you haven't seen before.

# INDEX

## ABOUT THE AUTHORS

**THE EDITORS OF SHARPMAN.COM** bring you
SHARPMAN.COM, the award-winning men's online community
providing men with "how-to" information on work, dating, grooming,
health and travel. Other books in THE SHARPMAN EDGE series
include:

**50 Great Dates for Any Budget**

**The Young SharpMan's Guide to Grooming:**
A How-To Book for SharpMen Ages 13 & Up

**How to Make a Pregnant Woman Happy:**
Quick & Effective Home Remedies for Over 60 of
Pregnancies Most Common Problems

For more information on SharpMan Press books and other
products, visit www.sharpman.com or contact SharpMan Press at:

SharpMan Press
11718 Barrington Court, No. 702
Los Angeles, CA 90049-2930
866-SHARPMAN (866-742-7762)
orders@sharpman.com